Yoganetics

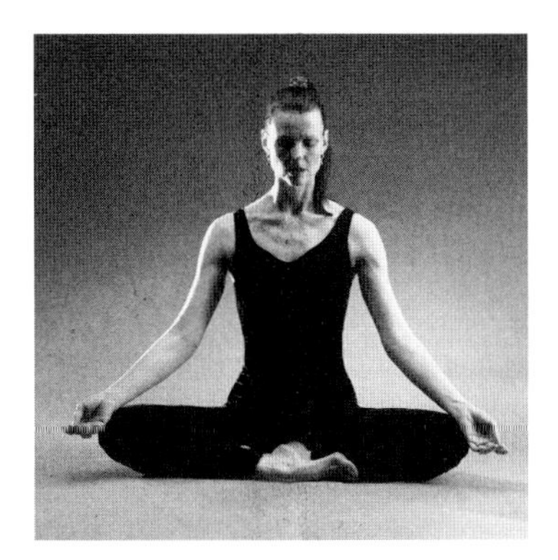

ALSO BY WYATT TOWNLEY

The Breathing Field: Meditations on Yoga
(poems by Wyatt Townley with art by Eric Dinyer)

Yoganetics: Relaxation and Basic Workout
(60-minute workout video)

Perfectly Normal
(poems)

Yoganetics

Be Fit,
Healthy,
and Relaxed
One Breath
at a Time

Wyatt Townley

For Students of All Levels and Traditions

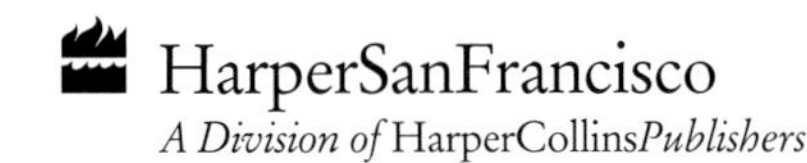
HarperSanFrancisco
A Division of HarperCollins*Publishers*

HarperCollins books may be purchased for educational, business, or sales promotional use. For information please write: Special Markets Department, HarperCollins Publishers, Inc., 10 East 53rd Street, New York, NY 10022.

HarperCollins Web site: http://www.harpercollins.com
HarperCollins®, ®, and HarperSanFrancisco™ are trademarks of HarperCollins Publishers, Inc.

FIRST EDITION
Designed by Joseph Rutt

Yoganetics® is a registered trademark with the United States Patent and Trademark Office.

Photography: Terry Weckbaugh, Image Quest

Library of Congress Cataloging-in-Publication Data
Townley, Wyatt.
Yoganetics : be fit, healthy, and relaxed one breath at a time / Wyatt Townley.—1st ed.
p. cm.
Includes bibliographical references.
ISBN 0-06-050224-X (pbk.)
1. Yoga, Hatha. 2. Breathing exercises. I. Title.

RA781.7.T65 2002
613.7'046—dc21
2002032701

03 04 05 06 07 RRD(W) 10 9 8 7 6 5 4 3 2 1

The author of this book is not a physician, and the ideas, suggestions, and instructions in this book are not intended as a substitute for medical counseling by a trained medical professional. For your safety, consult your doctor before beginning your practice. The author and publisher disclaim any liability arising directly or indirectly from the use of this book.

Not all exercises are suitable for everyone. This and other yoga/fitness programs may result in injury. Any reader assumes the risk of injury arising directly or indirectly from the use of this book.

An Invitation

But she was inside *the wonderful garden, and she could come through the door under the ivy any time, and she felt as if she had found a world all her own.*

FRANCES HODGSON BURNETT, *THE SECRET GARDEN*

Come as you are. No special gear or get-up required. Whatever the reason you opened this book, you are welcome here. Yoganetics is not the exclusive terrain of the young and thin, of contortionists, gymnasts, or dancers. It doesn't matter what kind of body you have or how many years it's been walking around.

Male or female, in shape or out, you are hereby invited to forget how you look. You are invited on a ride through your body, to find the secret path of breath and follow where it leads. As you travel the path within, your outer form will respond in wonderful, undreamt-of ways.

Just pull up a piece of floor and relax.

for Eric Beeler
and for my students
with gratitude

Contents

Preface

We come to this work "as is." Our immediate task is to become grateful for the body that has served us for a lifetime, exactly as it is, and exactly as it is not. We can transform and ultimately transcend the physical self, but first we must embrace it fully—especially the parts we don't like, the places we ignore, and the pockets of discomfort or pain.

How do you feel about your body? Whatever your answer, the body knows and responds in kind. Yoganetics provides a means of befriending the body, rendering it more responsive to training, and extending beyond this program into all aspects of life. The mind-body relationship is the crux of the matter in an age when contempt for the body has become a national pastime.

Our notion of beauty has been warped by models and celebrities who make up a fraction of 1 percent of the population and yet are inescapably everywhere, dominating billboards, newspapers, and televisions. This air-brushed minority has come to set the standard for the great majority. Ironically, these few who represent the gold standard aren't satisfied with their looks either, and many use drugs and surgery to get that way. So gleams the false ideal that we spend our lives measuring ourselves against.

Even dancers—those sylphs with perfect builds—don't like their physiques. In a recent *Dance Magazine* survey, just 23 percent of women (and 33 percent of men) were satisfied with their shape. And nearly 40 percent of female dancers think they are overweight, even though they rank *below ideal weight figures.*

It's time to reconsider our judgments. Whether we're thin, thick, short, or long, it's time to bless the package we find ourselves in, with all its wonders and difficulties. What would we need to give up in order to accept the body right now, in "as is" condition?

We would need to stop using someone else's idea of beauty and create our own. We would need to give up the effort our body enmity has required of us: the struggle to be what we're not, the resultant anger and devalued sense of self. And we would have to remember that who we are is greater than anything the body can contain—or attain. We are not our bodies. But let's treat them with the honor they deserve for bringing us this far, and learn to use them well.

Whatever our physical problems, they can lead to growth and grace. Cling to the difficult, urged the poet Rainer Maria Rilke. The difficulties will teach us to dance, if only we will let them. My own story exemplifies this process. For most of my life my body was a source of angst, until a litany of limitations and injuries brought me to this work, which changed everything.

As a toddler, I was so pigeon-toed and flatfooted that the doctor prescribed steel shoes and ballet training. At age thirteen, I shot up seven inches to become over six feet tall (that's seven feet *en pointe*) and over time developed a case of scoliosis to add to the mix. During the growth spurts that punctuated adolescence, I was never really sure where my body began or ended, so I became infamous for my stumbles and spills. I was a perfect klutz.

It was partly the challenge that dance presented to my un-ideal body that made me decide to pursue it as a career. Along the way I landed a wonderful role in Jim May's "D'Ambience." Instead of having one partner, I had twenty, and was tossed from one person to another, somersaulting and twisting every which way without ever touching down—until the very end of the piece, when my character died and was lowered to the floor. In dress rehearsal just before opening night, our nerves were high and our timing was off.

I was dropped from a height of about twenty feet and landed on my head. Though my spinal cord was intact, my neck was broken—and the doctors doubted that I'd ever dance again. They were wrong.

This crisis, like so many, was a (very) disguised blessing. Breaking my neck was the door to finding a way of working with the body that would heal instead of hurt. Recovering meant tracking down patterns of motion that led to pain and replacing them with smarter choices. With practice, the new choices would become reflexive and the healing process self-sustaining. Could such a simple, subjective approach work?

I returned to the earth for the answer. I literally sought my lowest level by lying on the floor and closing my eyes. In surrendering the fight with gravity, I learned how to exploit its power to realign the spine. By surrendering the sense of sight, I was able to find a new way of moving that didn't focus on how the body looked but on how it *felt*—a revolutionary experience that led to one revelation after another. I discovered how to source motion from the core, instead of wagging arms, legs, and head at their joints. Not only did my dance technique change, but my whole life was transformed. Yoganetics was born.

Gratitude is an appropriate beginning. I am grateful for the difficulties that ushered me here. This work saves me on a daily basis and has touched the lives of thousands who bring with them ailments ranging from arthritis to heart disease. These ailments are our keys to a new life.

Yoganetics stands on the shoulders of ancient yogic traditions that have been passed from body to body, generation to generation, for thousands of years. It has been influenced by many pioneers in the movement world, among them Martha Graham and Joseph Pilates. The work also owes a great debt to many in the fields of consciousness and the spine. But at its core, Yoganetics rests in the Japanese concept of *Hara,* the life-changing connection to one's center, as expressed magnificently by the German philosopher and psychotherapist Karlfried Graf Von Dürckheim.

Thanks to the State University of New York at Purchase for providing an early opportunity to pursue my twin passions of dance and writing. I am particularly grateful to these masters of movement, who helped me understand the physics of motion within my own body: Agnes de Mille, Irmgard Altvater, Tatania Dokoudovska, Jim May, Romana Krysanowska, Anna Sokolow, Kazuko Hirabayashi, Mette Spaniardi, Don Redlich, Finis Jhung, and Eric Beeler.

I am also grateful to the following editors of newspapers and magazines who believed enough in me to print my findings on the body: Brian Moss, Brenda White, Guy Flatley, Susan Benson, Warren Maus, Scott Cantrell, Steve Paul, Richard Philp, Gary Parks, Robert Johnson, David Sendler, Colleen Morton, and Jeanette Schoenlaub-Jackson.

Like life, publication is a mystery. This book would not exist had it not passed through the serendipitous line of hands that led like stepping-stones to your hands. Thanks to Eric Dinyer, the breathtaking artist who collaborated with me on *The Breathing Field: Meditations on Yoga,* for yoking me with the irresistible Sandy Choron, my dear agent and comrade, who placed this project in the lap of Renée Sedliar at Harper San Francisco, fellow poet and stellar editor.

For hosting the Yoganetics studio for the past dozen years, I am grateful to Unity Church of Overland Park and its devoted board and staff.

Special thanks to Rev. Greg Barrette, Lynn Barrette, Rev. Nancy Jerome, Kim Stryker, Caroline Krueger, Kent Baker, Leigh Smith, Jody Drake, Russ Swift, Roger Otterstrom, Dennis Klamm, Floyd Marshall, Ann Bowren, Tammy Joseph, Kathy Ganaden, Fred Albers, Charlie Carter, Janet and Rick Bacus, Alice Anderson, Charolette and Brad Goff, Leslie Anderson, Randy Gerard, Roger Davis, Mike Andes, John Mutrux, Melissa Mayers Lewis, and Rev. Mary Omwake for their ongoing support.

Yoganetics would not have translated so gracefully into book form without photographer Terry Weckbaugh of Image Quest. Thanks to Terry for his sense of adventure, masterful creativity, and patience with this perfectionist. Thanks also to book designer Joseph Rutt for his elegant grasp of the material.

No thanks can encompass my gratitude to my family, whose love helped bridge this work from body to page. I am grateful to my parents, Joanne and Russell Baker, for their generosity and counsel, and for the shoes that walked me here. Thanks to my husband, writer Roderick Townley, for his unswerving faith, his ability to move furniture in a single bound, and his visionary yet meticulous editing of numerous versions of this manuscript. Thanks to my daughter Grace for her empathy, for her insightful feedback, and for cheering me on through difficulty.

This book is dedicated to Eric Beeler, my brother in spirit, whose undulant yoga classes helped me break through the protective armor of my body to reveal the life force within. More than anyone I have ever danced with, reviewed, or seen on- or offstage anywhere, Eric was a clear demonstration of "poetry in motion." Since his passing, his spirit continues to guide and inspire.

To my students who have endowed me with the great privilege of learning through them, this book is also dedicated. Your own unfurling has furthered the evolution of this work and goes way beyond the body we use as our medium.

Finally, thanks to the spirit that underlies us, every move we make and breath we take.

Wyatt Townley

Introduction
Nobody's Home

"Colin," she began mysteriously, "do you know how many rooms there are in this house?"

"About a thousand, I suppose," he answered.

"There's about a hundred no one ever goes into," said Mary.

FRANCES HODGSON BURNETT, *THE SECRET GARDEN*

Where have we been? While we may have traveled the world, most of us haven't paid attention to our inner geography. As a result, we don't have access to the terrain within, from the tips of our ears to our little toes. Some of us live in our head, viewing the land south of the collar as practically a foreign country. Others of us cut ourselves off at the equator of the waistline and consider the lower body an altogether different hemisphere from the upper.

Wherever we have drawn our boundaries, we've divided the body into regions like a map. Some we live in, others we visit, and a few we've never heard of, much less speak the language. We're likely to favor the right side over the left, the upper over the lower, the front over the back, and the outside over the inside. Until we reintegrate our various parts and start to approach the body as a whole from the inside out, we're tourists instead of natives in our own skin.

To whatever extent we've cut ourselves off from the body, we relate to it as an object. Male and female, we objectify the body every time we regard it as a thing that follows commands (*Run faster! Lift the leg higher!*). The body is not a thing. It is a place, a living field of energy that most of us have never explored, much less called home.

"Yoganetics has been the key to my sense of living in my body again," says one practitioner. "It feels great, I feel great, I feel myself. The energy of the experience, the 'synergy,' is rejuvenating, invigorating, and relaxing all at once. I feel ageless and free when I get up and go back to my world. I feel like I'm doing something on a breakthrough level."

This sense of integration is not only exhilarating, it's readily available, but only if we're present enough to experience it. By the time we reach adulthood, many of us have virtually abandoned the body. It's as if someone gave us a mansion by the sea to spend our life in, but we never unpacked our bags. We're living out of a suitcase in the attic, peering out the little dormers of our eyes. Rarely do we venture down to the ground floor, much less enter the basement, where the plumbing is.

No wonder our culture is obsessed with sex. Besides providing the means to connect deeply with another person, sex invites us to go downstairs and occupy the locked basement, the netherworld below the waist. Making love may be the only opportunity we allow ourselves to listen and respond to our sensations. For many, it is the singular activity during which we feel truly integrated—mind, body, and spirit married in the moment.

But soon we're back to business as usual, above the belt and above the collar, cut off from the power within. We may try to compensate for this neglect by starting a fitness program. Guided by the desire to "get in shape" (an objectifying phrase if there ever was one), we approach the body like a garment we want altered. With the help of well-meaning experts, we start "cutting" new muscles in an endless, loveless cycle of weighing and measuring. We become fat-to-muscle ratios and body-mass indexes, pound by pound and inch by inch reducing our body to a set of stats.

Manufacturers have responded with a storm of products that take us still further from ourselves. We're now convinced we need machines, weights, steps, slides, balls, bands—the list gets longer each day—to work the body. Even the yoga world has joined in, with a blizzard of accessories all its own, from belts to bolsters. Ultimately, we're made to feel that we're not enough, that we must rely on things outside of us to be at home in the body—an untruth that preys on the insecure to generate millions for the ambitious.

Not only do we need props to "get fit," we need distractions from the props! Stairmasters are fitted with book stands. Televisions blare afront treadmill users, pulling us yet another step away. "Gym rats could spend half as much time in the gym if they were 100 percent focused on what they're doing," says Diana McNab, a sports psychologist who works with

Olympic athletes. And according to research at the University of Massachusetts, even the *psychological* benefits of exercise are reduced when the mind separates itself from the body.

Separation was the problem to begin with. The split is deepened in dance, yoga, and fitness studios that provide the most seductive diversion of all: the mirror. Dancers can become so addicted to the mirror that when they get onstage, they lose their bearings. The same goes for yogis as they attempt to transfer their training from the classroom to a home practice. The alignment they learned may be more visual than visceral.

Mirrors encourage us to approach the body from its surface, manipulating it like a suit of armor. In class, we mimic the shapes the instructor makes through visual cues. The process is *imitative,* imposing movement on the body from the outside in, and a world away from the highly *creative* process of discovering how to move organically, from within out.

Impositional training may seem normal, because the mirror probably got us to class in the first place. In fact, the mirror can play a role in helping us perfect form, but always at the expense of content. Because no matter how it may beguile us, the mirror is a wall. It separates us from who we are, what we are doing, and what we feel as we do it.

Nobody's home.

Beneath the Boredom

Underlying our thirst for distraction is fear. Superficially, we're afraid that without all the hoopla—without mirrors, television, and gadgets galore—working with our bodies is . . . boring. So runners chase down new routes. Instructors hunt up new steps.

The tedium factor has nothing remotely to do with routines. The problem is the approach. Exercise *is* monotonous, if it's approached from the outside in. Externalized movement is bound to become mechanical rather than deeply felt because it is something we are doing *to* our bodies rather than *through* them.

If we were merely to dive into our own experience of the body, we would never be bored again. It is that simple. There is a world within, every bit as exhilarating as the outer world with its bells and whistles. But to find it takes courage, because the real reason we seek distraction goes deeper than the fear of boredom. Without the paraphernalia, we'd have to face the fact that we're actually afraid of our bodies.

We don't want to get in there and listen to our breathing or locate our heartbeat. It's uncomfortably intimate. We're squeamish about sensations, afraid of pain, wary of pleasure. We're afraid of being messy, of being sweaty or bloody or sick. We are afraid of losing control. Being in the body can be scary, because the body is vulnerable. So we ignore it as much as possible. This is denial of the most basic kind, and the whole fitness world is based on it. Illness and injury are based on it. "I'm not doing this, I'm not feeling this, I'm not really here," is what we're pretending as we watch television from the treadmill or barrel through aerobics routines.

As we distance ourselves from the body, it in turn becomes desensitized. For many of us, months, sometimes years, of training are needed before we can even *find* our heartbeat without placing the hand on the chest. In this state of numbness, the body feels foreign—inarticulate and ungainly. It functions less well, so we pull further back.

For the first time in our nation's history, overweight people outnumber the slim. As we "put on" more weight and take up more space, we move still further from our core. The chasm between mind and body continues to widen until a crisis intervenes—or until the moment we turn toward home.

Eventually, the cry for help comes, although we may not recognize the message. To get our attention, the body may resort to sickness or injury, not unlike the child who misbehaves to gain the eyes and ears of a parent. In the realm of the body this tactic never fails. We catch a cold, we turn an ankle, or our back goes out, and suddenly we're forced to stop and focus on what we have neglected for so long.

Let's not wait for an injury or illness to bring us back to the house we abandoned. It's time for spring cleaning, to open the windows and doors and let light and wind move into every corner.

Coming Home

In this program, you will learn to live and move from the inside out. Like a child whose parents have been away, the body yearns for this kind of intimate attention. And it will respond to your nourishing care, first in feeling, and later in form.

We begin by returning to a playful, childlike state of exploring the body, starting from a point of innocence. The quotations that open each chapter will lead the way. These pearls, taken directly from children's literature, convey universal truths to discover in your practice. You will find the Secret Garden, the Golden Key, Neverland, Oz, and the Great Good Thing inside yourself.

Besides the twenty-motion beginner workout and the twenty-motion intermediate workout, this book includes twenty "experiments." Sprinkled throughout the text, these experiments are designed to train your powers of observation, using your body as a personal laboratory. The results are immediate as you catch yourself in the process of life and begin to replace old habits with smart ones. The more you spy on yourself, the more you'll discover about what it means to inhabit the body. In time, life itself becomes yoga.

Along the way, shifts in consciousness will occur as we make the transition from treating the body as a thing to *experiencing it as a place,* a place we can begin to call home. How does it really feel back behind the skin? How would it feel to pull our awareness down below the lines we've drawn at the collar and the belt? How would it feel to enter the lumbar chamber and the right fourth toe—and live from there? Imagine if we actually followed, rather than denied, our sensations during the day—or during a workout. Would we get anything done? Would we be in pain? Would we be in pure ecstasy?

And could we *stand* it?

Part One

The Power of Presence

One

The Plunge into Yoga

Then the Old Man of the Earth stooped over the floor of the cave. . . . disclos[ing] a great hole that went plumb-down.

"That is the way," he said.

"But there are no stairs."

"You must throw yourself in. There is no other way."

GEORGE MACDONALD, *THE GOLDEN KEY*

Yoga is a plunge into the self from which we emerge renewed and strengthened. Translated from the Sanskrit, yoga means "yoke," or "union." Its goal is unity—unity of mind and body, unity with self, others, and the spirit that runs through us.

Yoga will outlive us. It will outlive every body that has experienced its transformative power and every book that will be written about it. Long after Stairmasters and rowing machines pile up in landfills, yoga will continue to be passed from body to body, generation to generation. It has been happening for thousands of years. Today yoga has become the workout of choice among a growing number of executives, fitness mavens, and celebrities.

The reasons are clear: Yoga nourishes what needs to be nourished, strengthens what needs to be strengthened, stretches what needs to be stretched. Beyond the physical, yoga teaches us to attend to the whole and profound being that we are.

Form follows content. Look at the streamlined bodies of yogis to see the results of such integrative attention. What is unnecessary falls away. "My whole silhouette has changed," says one student. "I am now able to fit into my 'skinny clothes,'" says another. And what has been compressed unfurls: People routinely get taller.

What Is Yoga?

Yoga is a five-thousand-year-old living science begun in India that continues to evolve today. Some people wonder whether yoga will interfere with their own beliefs. Yoga is not a religion but a practical aid to living that can benefit anyone.

Generally speaking, yoga can be divided into four main paths: Karma yoga (the path of action), Bhakti yoga (the path of devotion), Jnana yoga (the path of wisdom), and Raja yoga (the path of science). Raja yoga is also called "the royal road," and Hatha yoga branches off from it to focus on the physical body.

Just as there are many wells to the river, there are many schools of Hatha yoga. Each has its own validity and leads ultimately to the same place—union of mind, body, and spirit. While there are as many approaches as there are teachers, basic similarities run through all techniques. Most classes include a series of postures, breathing exercises, and meditation. Students become still in each pose while relaxing and breathing deeply.

What Is Yoganetics?

Yoganetics is a form of Hatha yoga because it trains the physical body, but it departs from other techniques in several ways. First, Yoganetics (fusing "yoga" and "kinetic") extends yoga into motion. It is *transition*-based rather than *position*-based, fluid rather than static. Instead of emphasizing poses, we focus on the motion *between* them that creates and ultimately glues them all together. The postures themselves are secondary.

In Yoganetics the work is done on the floor, to realign the body without stressing the joints. Since balance is not an issue, we get to practice with the eyes closed, to foster a deep and integrating experience of where we really live. In that light, Yoganetics is gear-free, to remind us that everything we need is within us.

Most important, Yoganetics emphasizes content over form. Reversing the usual point of view, we shift the attention from the body's outer contours to the space and flux behind the skin. Through this life-altering shift, we can discover, one breath at a time, how to live and move from the inside out.

Why Motion?

Movement is the essence of life. It's what babies do in wombs, what stars do in space, what atoms do everywhere without cease. Life isn't a matter of taking a position and holding on to it as long as possible, though that's what many of us attempt. Life is blurry; it's what happens before and after the photos are snapped.

Of course, there's nothing wrong with making pretty pictures. Loads of dancers and models—and yogis—have made an art of it. But as yoga has migrated westward, it has become less a science in union than a competition in contortion, emphasizing results over process. Consider the full-page ad in a major publication: "Invitational Yoga Pose Off. $30,000 First Prize! Watch the world's best as they battle for prestige and cash!"

Instead of *pos*-ition, Yoganetics emphasizes *trans*-ition. Westerners tend to skip transitions. We are destination-oriented; we want to "get there." We get up, get dressed, get breakfast, get to work, get home, get to bed, and start all over again. Mostly, we're trying to be where we're not. What does this say about where we are?

Of course, as soon as we arrive, "there" becomes "here," and in short order we're off to the next place where we are not—yet. Because we prize the destination and discount the journey, we miss out on the scenery right in front of us. From the superhighway, it's hard to see into the trees whizzing by, or the secrets they shelter.

What happens *between* arriving and departing? Are we "there" when we're filling the gas tank or standing in line at the store? America's approach to fitness reflects this "destination consciousness." Although we want to "get fit," we don't actually want to work out! Afterward we feel great, but . . . during? This tendency shows up even in the supposed serenity of yoga class, when people rush themselves into postures the way they roar up to a stop sign. Both are jarring to the body, and both rob us of the journey, the "how" of motion, by focusing on the "where." What is the hurry? Where do we think we are going?

All too soon we'll be moving beyond the body. That's why it's so important, and so difficult, for us to slow down. Whenever we do, we paradoxically create *more* time. By literally slowing down—lowering heart rate, respiration, and blood pressure—we increase our rest between actions and extend the life of our organs, which get less wear and tear over the years.

Take the heart, a most suggestible organ. Think about something exciting, and it will speed up. Focus on something tranquil, and it will follow suit. The more you practice slowing down your inner tempo, the more responsive the heart will become.

Experiment: **Close your eyes and bring your attention inside your chest, just left of center. Ride the rhythm of your heartbeat. If you don't feel your heart beating from the inside, place a hand over the chest. Now, focus on the spaces between beats, with the idea of expanding these spaces.**

Don't worry if you don't feel your heartbeat, let alone slow it down. We'll be getting lots of practice throughout this book. Just as artists make the "negative space" between objects come to life, we can come to life in the many spaces of our lives. By letting go and anchoring in the here and now—even for a second—we can be reborn in the instant and experience the joy and innocence of who we are. Like the delicious space between heartbeats, life is made up of the moments between events.

So it is with yoga. In Yoganetics, we pay attention to the spectrum of movement between, say, bending and straightening a leg. Whether that leg ever gets straight is not important. It's *how* we move—not where we're going or how fast we get there—that matters. Our mission is to become dedicated to the journey rather than the destination. To accomplish this, we will learn to move in slow motion, distilling movement to its essence, while we experience what happens from deep inside the body. We will take the scenic route through the heart of the forest—and the forest of the heart.

Moving slowly is actually harder than moving quickly, requiring more lung capacity and a heightened ability to articulate the joints and muscles. People who race through life in high gear will find it challenging, but in Yoganetics the slowest person "wins." As we advance, our ability to sustain movement and breath increases, resulting in expanded lung capacity and range of motion as well as lowered resting heart rate and blood pressure. Slowing down is its own reward.

Dance is a wonderful metaphor for "journey" consciousness because the essence of dance is transition. Next time you're at a performance, pick out the best dancers. They aren't necessarily those who strike breathtaking poses. There are plenty of card-carrying professionals who hit their marks. But dance is what happens *between* poses, and the real artists are those who have learned to move *through* the positions in a stream of non-stop grace as one movement unfurls into the next.

French poet Paul Valéry said that a poem is never finished; it is finally abandoned. This applies to yoga. No motion or pose is ever finished; we are always in the process of arriving. There is always more room and breath—more space and time—to be discovered.

Why Floorwork?

The advantages of working on the floor are many. First, floorwork alleviates the stress on joints that comes from being vertical. As we surrender to gravity and release the accumulated tension of the day, muscles relax and bones fall into their natural alignment. We become neutral, a place from which we can undo a lifetime of harmful postural tendencies and begin to train the body anew.

We return to the earth for our lessons because we haven't yet mastered the art of standing on two feet, let alone running or hefting weights! It's no surprise we have an epidemic of back and joint pain among us. Many weight-bearing fitness techniques don't emphasize alignment, and so our less-than-perfect posture gets worse, not better, each time we work out.

By lying down we get to exploit, rather than fight, the force of gravity. Floorwork enables us to realign the spine and re-educate the muscles around that alignment to support us in daily life. With practice, this alignment transfers from the horizontal plane to the vertical as we sit, stand, and move—and life itself becomes a river of opportunities for conscious fitness (which we'll plunge into in part 3).

We are, after all, mostly fluid. Like water, we seek our lowest level. As we learn to move from the inside out, there is an underwater quality to our movement that carries us through all barriers and bumpy places. Our mission is to return to ourselves, to liquefy the body, transforming the stiff into the fluid. Like the tide, we respond to the pull of the earth and moon as breath rolls through us like a wave.

Working with the Eyes Closed

In a number of ways, the eyes have crippled the rest of the body.

Consider how you got where you are right now. Wherever you are and whatever position your body is in, you probably didn't smell your way there, or taste or feel or listen your way along. Unless you are blind, you saw your surroundings (the room, the beach) and negotiated your path around obstacles (desks, lawn chairs).

Our dependence on our eyes has led us to neglect the other senses, which in turn have grown less sensitive. In contrast, blind people have spent their lives sensitizing their other four senses. They *feel* their way through rooms, *smell* where the food is on the plate, *hear* the heels on the sidewalk before the doorbell rings.

By closing our eyes and removing our strongest sense, we strengthen the others. Suddenly we're aware of the smell of the carpet and the ticking of the clock. What's more, students report a greater ability to *feel* what's going on inside their bodies, heightening their sensuality (and sexuality).

Most important, working with closed eyes helps heal the split between mind and body—as well as the imagined separation between body parts. Instead of working arms and legs and hips and head and feet, we learn to move as one, anchoring all parts into the core, and rooting that center to the earth. The goal is integration.

Not unlike most issues, working with the eyes closed is largely a matter of trust. New students who feel unsure about sequence understandably keep their eyes open more than those who have studied for a while. But even veteran yogis may find themselves opening their eyes when they feel distrustful or stressed—for instance, during a motion they don't yet love. (The Groaner exercise is infamous for this.) We all share a tendency to return to the familiar when we are fearful. What does this stress response say about us and our outward-bound approach to fitness and the body? By and large, we're running scared.

That's fine. Eyes are terrific for negotiating around furniture and cars. But there are obstacles inside us that also need our attention. Closing the eyes and looking within is the first step to clearing a path in the body.

Gear-Free Fitness

Yoganetics is a gear-free zone. No equipment needed: no machines to maintain, no chairs to lug around, no steps or balls to store, no straps or bolsters to hunt down. We are returning to basics. This is self-contained fitness, and it goes everywhere we go—to Paris, to the beach, or to the floor of our office.

Just like a baby learning to crawl, we are going to begin our physical education all over again. We are going to discover muscles we never knew we had, and learn how to work one muscle group in opposition to another. By relying on gravity and the power of the breath to drive every motion, we will become fit from within out. Nothing added. A world gained.

Two

The Power of Yoga

"I think you'll find, Your Highness," said the girl with the dark blue eyes, "that distance isn't very important here."

RODERICK TOWNLEY, *THE GREAT GOOD THING*

The effects of yoga go far beyond the cosmetic. Yoga is therapeutic. It has been found to be both preventive and curative. Documented yogic benefits include a reduction in heart rate, blood pressure, stress, cholesterol, and blood sugar and a simultaneous increase in energy, lung capacity, digestion, and circulation.

The medical community is taking note. These days it's not unusual for doctors to recommend yoga for an array of ailments, and two-thirds of American medical schools now offer courses in alternative medicine. Research nationwide is gaining momentum with the establishment of the National Institutes of Health's Office of Alternative Medicine (OAM), and OAM's National Center for Complementary and Alternative Medicine (NCCAM).

Studies worldwide and an abundance of new data are bringing the yoga and medical communities closer every day. As evidenced by a growing body of research, yoga can be beneficial for arthritis, asthma, back pain, depression, fibromyalgia, cancer, AIDS, hypertension, and heart disease. (For more information on what's being learned about these conditions, refer to the Health Guide at the back of this book.)

Reversing the Stress Reflex

For people who think they are too busy to do yoga: Don't wait for your life to get less hectic to start this program. Yoganetics isn't another thing to add to your litany of "to-dos"—it will help you cope with the list. It's not another spoke in the whirling wheel; it is a hub activity. Hubs turn more slowly and connect all spokes to the core. People make a point of practicing Yoganetics *especially when they are busiest,* as a way to slow down and bring their lives into focus. "It has become a centering force in my days," says one student, an entrepreneur in the throes of a new business.

Stress is not a word our grandmothers used. Modern technology may have freed us from lugging pails of water from the river, but it has chained us to our desks. We may e-mail ourselves around the planet, but we have become cut off from our bodies and the world of nature. The unforeseen result: more stress.

How we manage it determines whether we live, get sick, or die. Stress underlies the process of illness, from headaches to heart disease. "Anywhere from 60 percent to 90 percent of visits to doctors are in the mind-body, stress-related realm," states Herbert Benson, M.D., a leading cardiologist at Harvard Medical School. With regard to chronic ailments, Benson says that "traditional modes of therapy—pharmaceutical and surgical—don't work well against them."

Yoganetics provides practical tools that can short-circuit the stress reflex, defusing tension while infusing the body with energy and power. The workout is truly a microcosm of life. What happens when we're under stress? What do we do when we find ourselves in an extremely uncomfortable position in life? That same thing will happen in an uncomfortable yoga position. Maybe the face tightens and the jaw locks, or the neck and shoulders clench. (One-fourth of the body's five hundred muscles are in the face and neck.) Such tension also affects our breathing—that is, if we don't stop breathing altogether!

We are about to discover our own stress reflexes, blow the whistle on them, and reverse those habits that don't serve us. Ours is the great work of life: finding the path and following it despite distractions, transforming uncomfortable positions into comforting ones, and learning to move through discomfort into peace. The techniques we learn here will permeate life at large, affecting how we breathe, sleep, sit, stand, make love, and handle conflict.

One woman consistently became upset when dealing with her ex-husband. "The last time I talked to him, I noticed I was becoming extremely tense and my neck and shoulders began to hurt," she recalls. "Within ten minutes of hanging up the phone, my chest started to pound and I had trouble breathing."

She lay down and did the path-breathing exercise in chapter 4. In just minutes, she says, "my whole body was relaxed, my chest no longer hurt, and I was 99 percent asleep."

Research shows that such techniques not only help lower blood pressure, heart rate, respiration, and other stress indicators but also influence the immune system, boosting the body's defenses against disease. Clearly, relaxation pays off. But we must learn *how* to do it.

Weight Loss

Overweight people outnumber the slim in our society. But heavy people—already at risk for joint damage—don't have to bounce themselves like balls to get fit. Research shows that using proper alignment *burns twice the calories* as slouching, according to Arthur White, M.D., former president of the North American Spine Society.

Alignment is all in the *how.* Most adults are hanging from their bones and degenerating their joints. As muscles learn to support the bones properly, a series of events occurs within. Muscles engage, energy is expended, more blood, oxygen, and fuel are delivered around the body, and more heat is produced, increasing our calorie usage.

With practice and over time, the proper alignment that we work on so assiduously in yoga translates to all aspects of life and promotes natural weight loss. Less fat means less fatigue. As the body learns to operate more efficiently, the energy level naturally rises. And the more energy we have, the more we feel like moving around, burning more calories. The process is self-sustaining.

Of course, weight loss has two components: calorie burning and calorie consumption. This program is also aimed at undoing the stress reflex that can lead to overindulging. One student, a nurse, lost twenty-two pounds over a twelve-week course. "Yoganetics has helped me learn to control stress," she says, "so I've stopped overeating."

Who Can Benefit from Yoganetics?

Yoganetics appeals to people at all points on the fitness spectrum. Students range from rank beginners to professional dancers, from teenagers to seniors, from back patients to insomniacs. If you can breathe, you can do Yoganetics. In fact, the program itself is an exercise in breathing.

A Note to Women

Our bodies undergo amazing transformations throughout life. We move from babyhood to girlhood to adulthood to old age, periodically ballooning up and down as we house other human beings. Then we disappear. What a ride!

Over the course of each month, our bodies are aswirl with news. When we're not growing babies, we tend to be preparing for (ovulating) or letting go of (menstruating) new life. These physical changes bring corresponding emotional sea changes. We create, let go, and bleed. Create, let go, and bleed. We're art in action.

Yoganetics offers an oasis during the process, even for those in the midst of a full-blown case of PMS. "Twice I've gone into class with menstrual cramps, and both times they were relieved," says one practitioner, a middle-school counselor. Working from the core brings our attention and breath right into the eye of the storm, and symptoms can dissolve in that place of power. The point is not to abandon the discomfort but to take its ride.

Likewise, women undergoing menopause find yoga can smooth the path. Yoga is used as an adjunct to hormone replacement therapy at centers such as Boston's Mind-Body Institute.

A Note to Men

When my daughter was five, she found out how to scare off the boys who chased her at school. "We just tell them we're going to play 'My Little Ponies,' and they run like mad!"

I once thought I only had to say one word to clear the room of men—not "marriage," but "yoga." That has changed! Lots of men fill our classes these days, but sometimes before they register their first question is: Are there are *other* men in the class?

"After a few weeks my flesh turned from a pillow into a mean, lean, dancing machine," says one convert, a musician. "I feel like a wild tree grown in a dry climate that has been transplanted to an oasis," says another.

Many find that Yoganetics helps them in sports. "My aim has improved in basketball," says a middle-aged writer, "because I can center myself and become calm. I've learned to breathe out when I shoot instead of holding my breath." Tennis and golf players are delighted to discover that this work can transform their game. And that's just the beginning.

Maybe you're afraid that you're not flexible enough to do yoga. It's true that women tend to be more elastic because of a few choice hormones floating around in them, but flexibility can be acquired. Muscles are pliable and respond to training—just as they can get stronger, they can also get longer. "For the first time since I was six years old, I can touch my head to my knees," says another male student.

That's fine and fun, but it's not important. This is not a contest to see who has the longest hamstrings. It's not the position that counts. *It's how you get there.* So relax. Compare yourself to no one. You are incomparable.

A Note to Athletes and Dancers

Your livelihood depends on your body's ability to move. Just as a violinist would take care of his Stradivarius, you must look after your own valuable instrument so it will serve you all your playing life.

"I could have never lasted as long as I did in the NBA without yoga," says former Los Angeles Laker Kareem Abdul-Jabbar. "Yoga became a kind of preventive maintenance. I found I wasn't as susceptible to muscle pulls or injuries as other players were."

"Clinically, people who stretch have a lower incidence of problems," says Peter Bruno, physician for the New York Knicks basketball team. Yoganetics is an excellent way to round out your training needs. After spending vigorous hours on your feet, non-weight-bearing exercise helps to iron out the kinks of the day—and realigns you for more efficient use tomorrow.

Yoganetics is gentle but very deep work. Moving with the eyes closed opens up an exotic new world to form-conscious athletes and dancers. It's like taking an able swimmer deep-sea diving for the first time.

A Note to People with Back Pain

This program is designed to change the habits that can lead to back pain. Over time, gravity and your own unconscious movement choices can hurt you. "Since taking this class, I've changed the way I stand," says one student. "I no longer have the lower-back pain I used to."

"At one time I could barely turn to the side to see if a car was coming," says another. "Now I can move freely without pain!" One woman who started Yoganetics with low-back pain has taken her tennis racket out of storage. Another can pick up her cat for the first time in years.

If you are having acute back pain—that is, if you are incapacitated or can't walk without feeling sharp, knifelike sensations—do *not* start this program until your back heals enough for you to function on your feet. Muscle spasm happens for good reason: The locking mechanism of a spasm limits your range of motion and helps prevent further injury. Respect your body's preventive "lock" by waiting for the spasm to release before beginning any exercise regime.

If you are functional (that is, out of spasm and acute pain when going through your day) but still feel occasional common backache, check with your health professional, then do the beginner workout, modifying with the Gentle Versions along the way.

A Note to Seniors

Some cultures revere their elders, but youth-obsessed America ignores them. Though this attitude is changing, the fitness world is still clearly the domain of young, glistening bodies bouncing to rock music.

That's a double whammy, to both joints and ears. Ninety percent of health clubs play music at volumes that can cause permanent hearing loss, according to research at Wichita State University in Kansas. To get fit, you don't have to hop around to ear-blasting music. Yoganetics is done on the floor to the sound of the breath within. Since it's non-weight-bearing, this work is easy on the joints and a natural choice for those of us who want to use them a few years longer.

Maybe you feel that your body is betraying you. More likely, you have abandoned it, particularly if you have chronic pain. It is time to come home again—to take the sheets off the furniture, pull open the drapes, and curl up in your favorite chair. If you have not been physically active, you may want to start with the Gentle Version modifications in the beginner workout. Let your body decide. As you become more familiar with the work, you can move from the modified to the regular beginner program, and progress to the intermediate level when you feel ready.

Thirty percent of the people I work with are seniors, and some are among my most advanced students. "I wish I'd found this twenty years ago!" is a common response, but it's never too late to begin. Whatever condition you're in, get ready to change. Your body will respond to this training because you will be attending to it in a new and deeper way.

Doing this work is as simple as falling into bed at night: We're all just lying down, closing our eyes, and taking a remarkable trip.

Three

Inhabiting the Body

"I lay a long time, and the moonlight got in at every tear in my clothes, and made me feel so happy—"
George MacDonald, *The Back of the North Wind*

Experiment: Next time you go to a big party, sweep the room with your gaze. Chances are you'll spot one or two people who stand out in the crowd. The air around them feels charged, and people feel energized just being near them. The room feels different when they enter or leave. What is it about them that draws your attention?

Hollywood calls it the "x" factor. It isn't what people wear or how good-looking they are. You can spot it at the theater in the chorus of a musical. All the performers are attractive and dressed exactly alike, but, for no apparent reason, certain ones stand out. They may not be the best dancers, they may not be the tallest in the cast, and they may be in the back row of the crowd. But something about them is different, and you can't take your eyes off them.

They don't call it stage *presence* for nothing. Stage presence is simply the quality of being present in the body in the moment. The more fully a performer occupies his or her body, the more palpable the presence. Those who act from the neck up, who remain "in their head," give a small and intellectual performance. Those who get down below the belt discover an energy that is bigger than they are. Even diminutive actors can look larger than life because of the degree to which they are *present.*

Of course, we don't have to be onstage to be fully present. But we have to be exactly where we are, instead of resisting the "now" by rerunning the past or projecting the future. Remember the last time you laughed out loud when you were alone? Something surprised you, and you were overcome. Or the moment you caught sight of someone you loved. The light changed; colors got clearer; sounds got richer. For that second you stopped living in the past, chewing its food and doing its laundry. You came home to the present and simply responded.

Life is full of such surprises, big and small. We may think we know what is going to happen in the next five minutes, and what won't happen. We don't. The phone rings; the doorbell rings; the body rings with life-changing news.

There are many roads to now, many attention-focusing meditation techniques to help us arrive where we are. Returning to the body never fails. It's simple, it's steadfast, and it responds to our attention by behaving better.

Closing your eyes and dropping down inside will anchor you. Below the waist is a sacred place. Deep in the cave of the belly, in the actual center of the body, you are going to settle in and make yourself at home. The more you return here, the more established the core will become. And the more established your core, the more connected you will feel to your life force as you discover the solace and safety you have sought, but never found, in the outer world. Here is a refuge in the midst of you, and it goes where you go. As you learn to live and move from the cave, the view just gets better and better. (We'll be taking a closer look at this phenomenon, called *Hara,* in the last chapter.)

Within you is a boundless energy, yours for the tapping. When you find it, you can't help yourself: You radiate through every pore. This is your natural state, over which layers of fatigue and world-weariness have settled. These layers are simply veils to be peeled off and thrown to the wind.

"I always leave the class feeling renewed, physically more unified, and with a lighter heart," says a student. One of these days we're going to take before-and-after photos, because people look very different after doing Yoganetics. They glow.

Practicing the Presence

The following exercise will help you to be more present in your body and to dive into your own reservoir of energy. Some call it a "guided visualization." I call it a voyage. We will be putting the body into a poetic state, using the power of metaphor.

This voyage precedes every Yoganetics workout. Before we do anything with the body, we must first *un*do, letting go of accumulated stresses and habits that interfere with our natural flow and would impede yoga or physical training of any kind. Bringing our consciousness into every forgotten corner and crevice is the first step in reclaiming ourselves.

As you mentally move through the body, you'll discover lots of little places where you have been harboring tension. That's an excellent sign, indicating that you are really present, instead of avoiding what's going on inside you. Treat your tensions as buried prizes you are unearthing, transforming your "tension hunt" into a treasure hunt (more on this in chapter 8). Your job is to bring the attention into the tension and watch what happens. As you move in, tension moves out.

The voyage takes about ten minutes but can be lengthened or shortened as needed. Some people use it as a morning meditation to launch the day. Some practice at night to help themselves sleep. Others use it as a relaxation technique before a presentation.

You'll be taking the ride in Corpse Pose, so named because it requires nothing of you but that you stop fighting gravity and allow the earth to support you. With practice, you will be able to take the tour in any position, in any place. People do it secretly at their desk, in the grocery line, or in the wings of the theater.

Just follow along, making your way through the body as you explore the space behind your skin. Nature imagery is used as a means of vivifying the landscapes within and reconnecting you with the restorative power of the natural world. If you don't feel what is suggested, experience whatever you do feel. If some of the images don't make sense to you, just play along and visualize them as fully as possible. And don't be surprised if unexpected emotions surface. Such feelings may have been locked inside the body and need to be released. Accept them, be grateful for them, then gently let them go as you return to the ride.

Above all, be patient with yourself and this remarkable process. If you like, read your way through the voyage before actually taking it. Just browsing through the suggestions will go a long way toward releasing tension. If you have a friend at hand, you can give the ride to each other. Better yet, become your own guide by reading the italicized parts into a tape recorder. Then you can practice at leisure or at bedtime. Speak each word slowly, pausing to breathe after each sentence and at the end of each paragraph.

Set aside a few minutes now. Turn down the lights, turn off the phone, lie down, close your eyes . . . and get ready to wake up.

The Inner Voyage

A Guided Tour of Your Body

Lying on your back, close your eyes and relax. Let the limbs stream out from the body: legs hip-width apart; arms 45 degrees from your sides, palms facing the sky, ready to receive. (If this position becomes uncomfortable at any time, just bend your knees and plant your feet on the floor.) [pause]

Forgetting what you look like, come down inside the body and start to feel what you feel like, on the level of pure sensation. Sense the floor beneath you—its texture, its temperature, and the support it offers. [pause] *Let the crown of the head and the tailbone drift in opposite directions.* [pause] *Lengthen the distance between your sitting bones and your heels.* [pause]

Rest. Unwind the muscles that wrap the bones, and let the bones fall into the earth. Allow the joints to open—the spaces between bones through which light is flowing. Surrender the weight of the body to gravity. Let go. The earth will catch and cradle you. [pause]

Imagine that your spine is a river. As you visualize this river flowing between your head and tailbone, become aware of the space behind the waist and the space behind the neck. Drop your chin and lengthen the back of the neck and the back of the waist, so the river can course freely through you. [pause]

Drop the shoulders away from the earlobes. Bring your attention up inside your head, where most of us spend most of the time. Come back behind the face, and feel its features from the inside. Let go of that expression you have worn for so many years. Let the brow slide open.

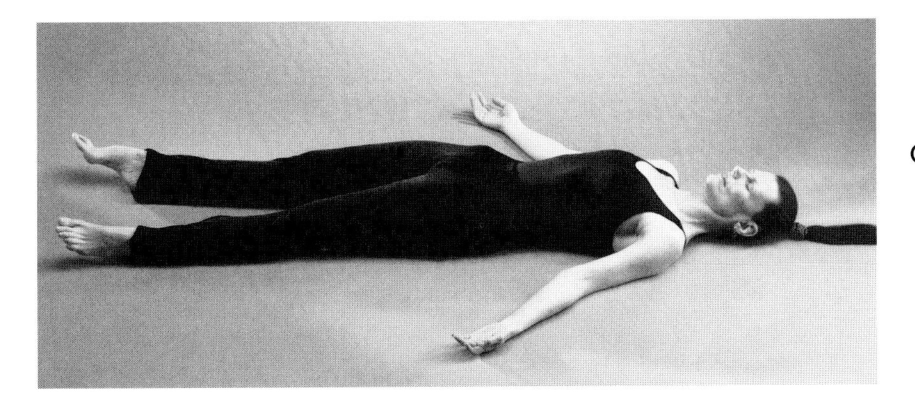

Corpse Pose

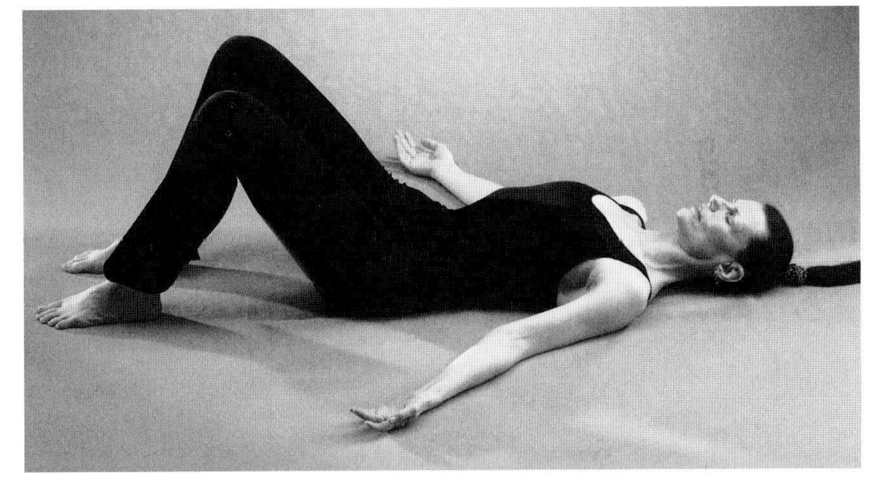

Modified Corpse Pose

Watch the eyebrows sail off to opposite horizons. Uncoil the little muscles around the eyes. Let the eyes soften and the eyelids drape gently over them, their corners streaming out like banners in the wind. [pause]

The cheeks go slack, poured over the cheekbones like liquid satin. Loosen and drop the jaw. If the jaw is really dropped, the lips will separate. As the lips part, they begin to relax and thicken. Let the tongue sleep in its deepening bed. [pause]

Visualize a vast horizon between your eyebrows and watch it expand. Find another horizon between your temples, and allow it to unfurl. Yet another horizon between your ears is unrolling in two directions. [pause] *Now imagine an opening at the crown of the head. Through this opening, light pours into the globe of your expanding awareness.* [pause]

Inhale and let the wind and light sail through the canal of the throat. Stream on across the collarbones, gushing through shoulders, down the long canals of the arms into the wrists. Take a moment to see if you can feel your radial pulse beating here as you ride the inner rhythm behind where the watch has lived. If you don't feel your pulse, experience what you do feel here in the wrists. [pause]

Now move on into the hands, palms, and fingers. Let go of everything you have ever held—steering wheels, coins, keys—and notice what the hands are really holding. You may become aware of a tingling sensation, an effervescence moving from behind the palm into the space on the other side of the skin, like steam rising off a whirlpool. Focus on what you feel—if it's tingling, fine. If not, what? [pause]

Returning to the source of your pulse, find the island of the heart, just left of center in the chest, between the front and back of the body. Beaching yourself on the shore of the heart, let yourself sprawl and bask here. Explore its shape, its size—slightly bigger than your fist—then let the light slide into it, allowing the fist of your heart to open. [pause]

See if you can feel your heart beating from the inside. If not, place your hand over the chest. Rest, and simply ride your own rhythmic embrace.

As you become aware of your inner rhythm, move into the space between heartbeats. Notice how this space begins to expand, and the heart slows down. Take your time. [pause]

And take your space. From the organ of the heart, expand on into the heart center, in the middle of the chest, between sternum and spine. Feel the light radiating from this place, as if the sun were rising right here in your heart center. Let the light beam out in all directions and all dimensions—forward, backward, sideways, and diagonally—streaming beyond the body into infinity. [pause]

Now let light slide downward through you, illuminating the path of the spine—each vertebra a stepping-stone that leads you through the cage of the ribs, across the bridge of the waistline, and on into the great cave of the belly and pelvis. The light flows into every corner of the cave, shining away all darkness. [pause]

In this safe and sacred place, find your center of power, the exact midpoint of your body. It's just above the pubic bone—very low—and just in front of the spine—very deep. Here is your gravitational center, halfway between the head and toes (or as a shortcut, between navel and pubis), halfway between the left and right side of the body, and especially, halfway between the front and back. [pause]

From this depth, drop anchor into the earth. Feel the pull of gravity from your own gravitational center, like a long umbilical cord that connects your core to the earth's core, belly to belly. [pause]

Anchored here, and nourished by this connection, watch as the light flows on throughout the hips, swirling in their open sockets, around backside through the buttocks and the bones they surround, and underside through the pelvic floor and all the organs it supports, including the genitals, working together in harmony. [pause]

Streaming on into the long tunnels of your legs, see if you can feel your thighs equally, left as well as right. If you experience one more clearly than the other, pay attention to the neglected side. Let the light whoosh on through the open knees, plashing down shins and calves, spilling through ankles into feet and toes. [pause]

Feel the entire body now, fully inhabited from head through toenails, lit from within. [pause] *You occupy the lower body as brightly and clearly as you do the upper, legs as well as arms, feet and hands equalizing.* [pause] *You inhabit the left side of the body as fully as the right.* [pause] *You're as aware of the back half of the body as you are of the front half.* [pause] *And you are conscious of the inside of the body as well as its familiar surfaces.* [pause]

Focusing on the soles of the feet now, see if you notice a tingling sensation in the bottoms of your feet. [pause] *If not, feel whatever you do feel here.* [pause] *Now tune in to both the soles of the feet and the palms of the hands, as if they were four quadraphonic speakers through which vibration is passing. It's easiest to sense this energy in the palms and soles, though it's coursing through us all the time.* [pause]

Sheer energy bubbles upward, as if the body were a great glass of champagne. We're going to reverse our journey now. On the ride back to where we started, see if you can visualize and feel this effervescence rising upward through you. Along the way, if you discover any barriers to the flow of energy, just ride your way through them and watch them dissolve. [pause]

[Read slowly] *Tuning in to the soles of the feet now, invite this tingling energy to rise upward through the ankles,* [pause] *fizzing up through the lower legs and knees,* [pause] *and coursing through the tunnels of the thighs.* [pause] *Let it bubble upward through the pelvis,* [pause] *swirling through the pelvic floor, buttocks, hips, and the cave of the belly,* [pause] *sizzling up through the wind tunnel of the torso,* [pause] *and into the heart center.* [pause] *Feel the heart center tingling, connected from the soles upward by this rising energy wash.* [pause]

Moving from the palms of the hands now, the effervescence courses upward through the wrists, [pause] *the long channels of the arms,* [pause] *through the shoulders,* [pause] *across the collarbones, and into the heart center. Take a moment to feel the tingling strongly in the area of the heart.* [pause]

From the heart center the sensation rises upward through the open throat and on into the head, streaming out through the crown, beyond each and every hair. [pause]

Feel the free flow of energy throughout the entire body now, from your soles through your crown. [pause] *From the bottom up, the body is awash with a rising effervescence, recharging in a living field of energy.* [pause] *Every limb, every muscle group, every organ, and every cell are humming together in response, a universal, harmonizing vibration that underlies everything you thought you were.* [pause] *Remain in this champagne state for as long as you like.*

How do you feel? If you've just taken the voyage, you may have gone somewhere that you never knew existed. Possibly you discovered some sunken treasure. Maybe you had trouble concentrating or felt silly doing the visualization. Whatever happened to you is right. If you felt euphoric, you're normal. If you felt distracted, you're normal. It's *your* voyage, and it will change each time you take it. So whatever you felt—or didn't feel—isn't important. Just take the ride, and let it lead you.

It's best at first to set aside a regular time and place for the voyage every day, to honor it as an occasion. With practice, the position itself will cue your body to release, and the "relaxation response" will become reflexive. You'll know this reflex has been established when you take Corpse Pose and discover your tension gushing out, your head blooming open, your bones waterfalling into place, and your body naturally recharging. Like a pebble tossed into still water, such a reflex becomes "contagious" and spreads out in every direction, rippling to all distant shores of the self and others.

Over time your body is going to become a familiar yet exotic place to live. You won't want to stay above the belt or above the collar anymore. You will be present inside yourself, with as much access to those distant toes as you now have to your fingers. You will gain entrance to all the little locked doors within that have been off limits for so long.

And you will fling them wide to the forces of light and wind.

Four

The Path of Breath

Mary was at the window in a moment and in a moment more it was opened wide and freshness and softness and scents and birds' songs were pouring through.

"That's fresh air," she said. "Lie on your back and draw in long breaths of it. . . . "

. . . and he did as she told him, drawing in long deep breaths over and over again, until he felt that something quite new and delightful was happening to him.

FRANCES HODGSON BURNETT, *THE SECRET GARDEN*

Spring cleaning has begun. We've pulled open the blinds and let in the light. Now it's time to open the windows and let in the wind.

Breath is life. We can go weeks without food, days without water, but without breath we die in minutes. You'd think we'd pay attention to so vital a function. But since breathing is automatic, most of us haven't taken time to ride the wind behind our skin.

Deep inside the body, along the front of the spine, is a secret path the breath can follow. This path connects two potent yogic centers—the power center in the pelvis and the heart center in the chest—bringing love to the power and power to the love. For so many of us who have cut ourselves off at the waist, traveling the path reunites the long-lost lower body with the upper body. Breath is the thread that sews us back together.

Path breathing is the core of Yoganetics. It is the *content* of every exercise, whether the *form* involves lying down, sitting up, kneeling, being prone or upside down. Whether you are working the left or right side, moving slowly or quickly, all you're really doing is traveling and deepening the path within.

The benefits of path breathing go way beyond survival. To breathe, or "inspire," derives from the Latin root *spiritus*. By bringing the unconscious activity of breathing to consciousness, we can experience body, mind, and spirit as one. Conversely, when we cut ourselves off from the breath, we disconnect from the power within.

Experiment: **Next time you're stressed or frightened, become aware of your breath. Do you find yourself breathing shallowly or holding your breath? What happens to its rhythm—is it smooth or staccato?**

Stress affects the way we breathe. The breath may get shallow or bumpy—if we're breathing at all. In any case, we aren't getting the oxygen we need. But the equation works both ways: Just as our mental state affects our breathing, *breathing can affect our state of mind.*

We carry within us a path to tranquillity that returns us to our natural state, as reflected in lower blood pressure and heart rate. "Five minutes of path breathing lowered my blood pressure from 132/83 to 114/64," says a male in his sixties, "and my pulse from 74 to 64." One woman with high-normal blood pressure developed "whitecoat syndrome" and recorded higher numbers in the doctor's office. "Now I do the breathing and have a 'good' reading," she reports.

It's all in the training. Through path breathing, you can learn to reverse your own stress reflex—and a score of stress-related problems from headaches to insomnia. Awakened by a loud noise in the night, one person noticed, "I was holding my breath. I started path breathing, and after four breaths I was back asleep again, just by concentrating on the path and nothing else."

Breathing the path not only relaxes the body but clarifies the mind. "I was trying to do three things at once," said an IRS auditor juggling angry phone calls. "Path breathing made me think more clearly. I was just amazed!"

After just five minutes of practice, a college student felt "a great, deep relaxation, a shedding of the day, so to speak." Afterward she did two hours of studying and experienced, to her surprise, greater focus "as well as an increase in retention of the material." Beyond the immediate mental and psychological benefits, path breathing expands lung capacity, improves digestion and circulation, and tones the abdominals. What more incentive do we need?

How Not to Breathe

As weird as it sounds, most of us have forgotten how to breathe properly. In fact, we have actually managed to *reverse* the natural breathing process.

Experiment: Here's a quick way to check your breathing pattern: Pull in your stomach. Now, did you inhale or exhale as you did this?

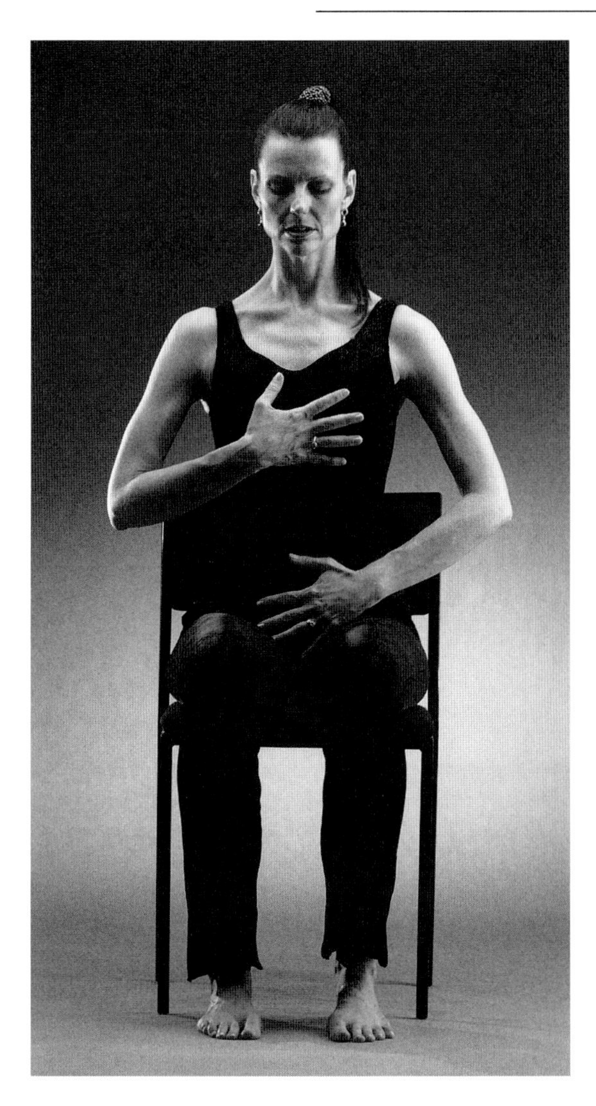

Which hand moves?

If you inhaled, you're like most of us misguided adults. Somewhere along the line, whether in gym class or the military ("Chest out! Shoulders back!"), we learned to suck in the belly while inhaling. This unfortunate habit creates tension in the shoulder, neck, and jaw muscles and may ultimately shorten the spine. We're going to undo all that. But first, another test.

Experiment: Place one hand on the chest and one hand on the low abdomen. Now inhale. Which hand moves?

If your upper hand moved, you (like most people) are breathing shallowly. We tend to take in about a pint of air per breath, barely filling the top of our lungs and using less than 20 percent of our three-quart capacity.

To learn how to breathe again, a great shift is required: from shallow to deep, from above the waist to below, from chest to abdominal breathing. It's another world down in the pelvic cavity, an entirely different hemisphere. To get there, we must be willing to move from the safety of the familiar to the untraveled unknown.

Our guides are everywhere. For starters, take a refresher course from a child (or any mammal, for that matter). Next time you spot your baby or pet asleep, take a good look at the tummy. Go to the zoo and watch the sea lions. All these sensible creatures allow their bellies to *expand* on the inhalation.

What happened to us? The very notion of expanding the abdomen goes against our culture. Many of us tend to contract our abdominals in an effort to look thin, a habit that may actually be counterproductive. If you half-hold your tummy in all day, your muscles can get locked into position, unable to be either stretched or strengthened.

To breathe properly, you'll have to let go of the fear of looking fat. Paradoxically, it is only when you relax the abdominals, allowing them to stretch on the inhalation, that you can more effectively work those same muscles as they contract organically on the exhalation. Breathing then becomes an act of tummy toning.

The Anatomy of Breath

Every breath is an act of purification. Each inhalation delivers essential oxygen to the body, and each exhalation releases waste in the form of carbon dioxide. To accomplish this deep cleansing, we rely on one of our most intriguing muscles: the diaphragm. After the heart, it is our most active body part.

The very word—*dia*, "across," and *phragm*, "partition"—speaks for itself. Some twelve to fifteen inches in diameter, its sheetlike structure stretches horizontally between the chest cavity and the abdominal cavity, serving as a floor for the heart and lungs and a ceiling for the liver, stomach, and spleen. In path breathing, the diaphragm moves vertically, massaging adjacent organs and stimulating digestion and circulation. During inhalation it lowers, providing the lungs with room to expand while creating a vacuum that draws air in.

Since the abdominal muscles are interwoven with the fibrous tissues of the diaphragm, they go along for the ride. "The descent of the diaphragm raises the pressure in the abdominal cavity, and as it ascends, the abdominal muscles are toned," wrote the late, great pioneer of posture Mabel Elsworth Todd in *The Thinking Body*. Further, she says, "Reciprocal action between the diaphragm and the abdominal muscles is so marked that where there is a loss of tone in the abdominal muscles . . . the action of the diaphragm may be seriously disturbed." In other words, not only does proper breathing strengthen abdominals, but strong abs foster better breathing. The ideal symbiotic relationship!

Often this process is called "deep breathing" or "complete breathing." I find those words too abstract. (Just watch what happens when you ask someone to take a "deep" breath: the shoulders and chest go up, telltale signs of shallow breathing.) Others speak of "abdominal breathing" or "belly breathing," but these phrases reflect the end and not the means. "Path breathing" enables us to experience the journey of the breath more deeply—not just its destination, but its increasingly long and mesmerizing ride.

Finding the Path

The path is an open secret. You can find it in the landscapes of Maurice de Vlaminck, the twentieth-century Fauvist artist. You can find it in Walt Whitman's "Song of the Open Road" and Robert Frost's road less traveled. The path is within the body as well, invisible but palpable. "Each one goes on this Path without moving his feet. . . ." says *The Eternal Verities,* a theosophical text. "This Path lies right in our own home, and wherever we go forth from home to any other place. This Path is in our schoolroom, at work and at play, every day and all the time, both awake and asleep."

To find the path, try this one-minute exercise.

Lie on your back with legs straight or bent, and place your hands on your low belly between the hipbones. Close your eyes and relax. Now focus on the heart center, in the middle of the chest between sternum and spine. Imagine you can breathe directly from this place. Inhale and follow the wind downward, filling the belly and hands, which rise softly. Exhale and feel your belly falling as you visualize the wind flowing back up the spine and pouring into the heart. Follow the breath slowly up and down the spine in this way for a minute, feeling the path unfurl through you.

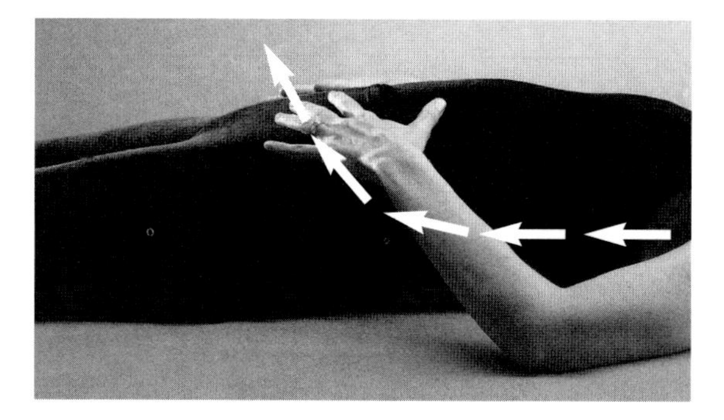

Feel the downward motion of the inhalation as it fills the belly.

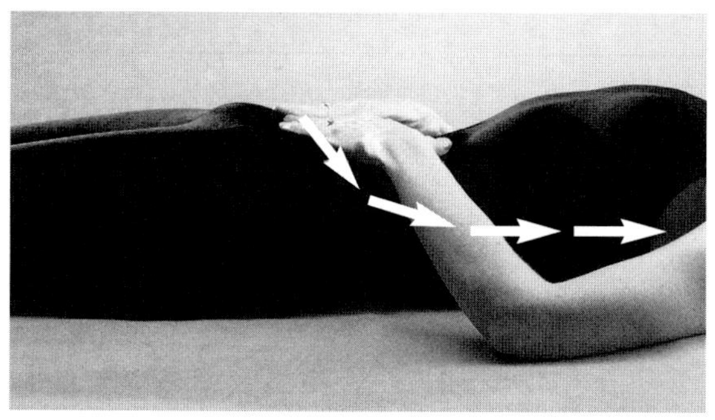

Feel the belly fall and follow the exhalation along the spine.

How do you feel? At first the path of breath may feel bumpy, with little fits and starts. Just keep going. The wind will overcome any obstacle it faces, just as water smoothes pebbles in the streambed until they disappear.

Maybe you found yourself running out of air, gulping in and blowing out as if there's a dearth of breath. Not so! In fact, you have an abundance of it—far more than you are using. To slow down the inner wind, simply reduce the size of your wind tunnel. Visualize a slender straw or tube along the front of the spine, through which an endless stream of air is flowing. Sip your breath like a drink through this secret straw and watch it slip up and down through you. In time, as your lung capacity grows, you can expand the size of your straw back into the wind tunnel of your torso and eventually beyond the body altogether.

When you are comfortable path breathing for one minute, increase to five. Once you have established the path in Corpse Pose, try it sitting. The path turns vertical when you're upright: The inhalation falls down the front of the spine deep into the well of the belly, and the exhalation rises like a fountain through the heart. Eventually you will be able to find the path at any time, anywhere, in any position or circumstance.

Stress as a Door

The next time you find yourself frustrated or upset, try to solve this math problem.

Experiment: In the midst of a stress "fit," breathe your way through the feeling. Travel the path and count your breaths. How many did it take you to recover?

Sometimes a single breath is all that's needed. Sometimes it may take thirteen, or thirty-four, or more than a hundred. It doesn't matter. What matters is that you use the path and remember that it's always there to move you across the bridge from stress to peace.

Where might you find this stress-busting technique useful in your life? Start small and practice your way to handling bigger conflicts. Travel and tally the path when you're running late for anything. Count your breaths with the telemarketer who interrupts your dinner. Practice with the slow waiter, the indifferent clerk, and the late friend. Standing in line offers terrific path-finding opportunities, whether you're at the store, the bank, or the theater.

Traffic jams also provide good practice periods, although we need to keep the eyes open! "If drivers were required to take Yoganetics," says one man, "maybe there would not be so much road rage."

Doctor appointments and procedures are perfect occasions to travel the path. "I do much better on unpleasant doctor exams," says one woman. "By path breathing and going within myself, I came through the last two tests with flying colors. It was so great not to be scared."

One of my favorites is the dental chair. I now view a visit to the dentist as a mini-vacation, an oasis from the day, since path breathing transformed me from a squeamish squid of sensitivity into a model patient.

Once we have added path breathing to our tool belt, our biggest challenge is to remember it's there so we can use it as needed. We all forget how powerful we are. Something as simple as wearing a rubber band can help us remember to breathe the path throughout the day. Or post a note on the mirror, the computer, the phone, wherever your eyes return on a regular basis. Hook it into your daily routine—whenever you sit down to a meal, pause at a stoplight, or use the bathroom.

One student came up with a wonderful reminder. Every time she went through a door, she would start breathing the path. Think of all the doors you have moved through today, beginning with your bedroom door, the bathroom door, the front door, and on through the many entrances and exits you unknowingly have made. Each door is a cue to follow the path.

Let's take that one step further and view the stressor itself as a door. Stress is neither good nor bad; it's just a door. Beyond the door lies the path, waiting in the wind.

Path Meditation

You now have the makings of a simple, organic meditation that can serve you for the rest of your life. We use it at the beginning of every Yoganetics workout: first, a few minutes to tour the body, then a few minutes to ride the wind along the path. It doesn't have to take long, and its clarifying effects will ultimately save you time.

In the words of a longtime practitioner, "Body and mind seem to slide or ooze into one force, one being." Taking the voyage and feeling the path unroll through you is an exquisite experience to give yourself. Be generous.

You don't have to practice in any special position, though lying in Corpse Pose is easy, and sitting cross-legged is traditional. You can practice secretly at your desk. No one has to know what you're doing. This form of meditation requires no occult initiations or special knowledge of Sanskrit. It is a visceral, literally sensational way to discipline the mind and refresh the body.

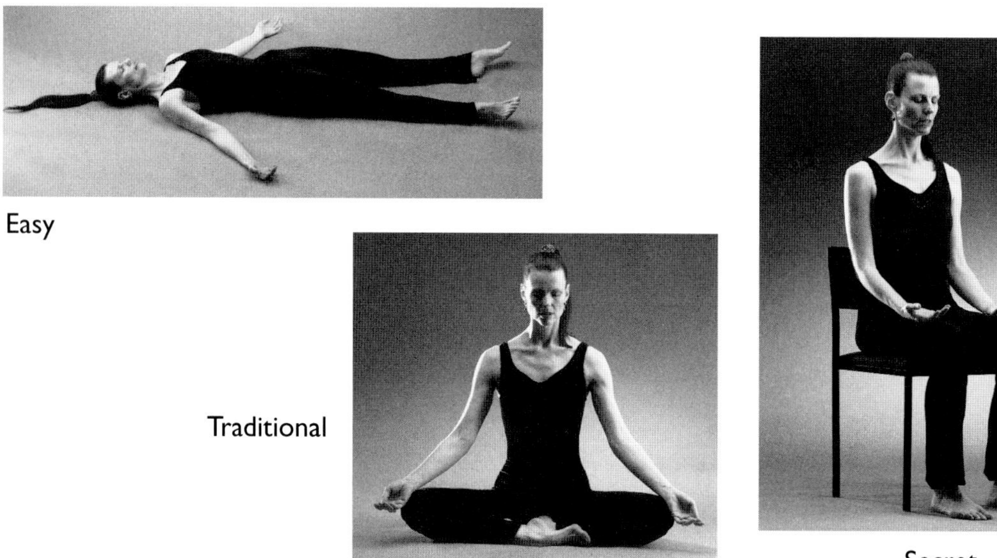

Easy

Traditional

Secret

Once you've cleared the path you need to *use* it to keep it open. Set aside time every day—even one minute—for your secret journey. Soon five minutes will fly by, then twenty. The length of time is less important than the quality of your attention. Still, you may run into obstacles along the way that block your passage. That's part of the process. On any path weeds spring up, trees topple down, and spiders spin their sticky webs. Don't get discouraged. As in the legend of Sleeping Beauty, you may have to cut your way through thorns on the path to the castle. The journey is worth it. Stay your course and keep going.

The Ocean in the Shell

In time, the path will become so well established that you will travel it without thinking, even as you sleep. Then you can add yet another sense to enrich the voyage. Some advanced students wear earplugs to help them hear the sound of the wind blowing through them.

Experiment: As you read this, press your index fingers over your ears. You are turning down the white noise of the outer world to hear the sound of the ocean inside the shell of your body. Now travel the path. Listen as your breath flows far away into the belly and back to the shore of your heart again. Close your eyes and let the tide roll through you.

Wherever you are, the pathway is—deepened and enriched by every breath you take. Let the world dote on outer form while you attend to the content. Rely on it and return to it when you get lost. The path of breath will lead you home.

Part Two

The Workout

Five

Preparing for the Workout

"It doesn't happen all at once," said the Skin Horse. "You become."

MARGERY WILLIAMS, *THE VELVETEEN RABBIT*

Each Yoganetics workout comprises twenty exercises and lasts about an hour. You do not need to practice every day. Every other day is optimal, but working out twice a week (evenly spaced, say Mondays and Thursdays) is enough for the technique to start "sticking." Some people schedule a regular time and don't vary from it. Others discover the best time as each day progresses. Some prefer working out in the morning to launch the day; others do it at night to unwind after work; still others like to recharge themselves during lunch hour. Whatever works for you is right.

What You'll Need

Yoganetics is done in bare feet and comfortable clothes that will let you move. You don't need a special outfit, gear, or equipment of any kind. All you need is a piece of earth big enough to lie down on and sprawl in all directions. A carpet makes a terrific workout area. If you have a hard floor, you might want to use a bathmat or exercise mat so your spine won't bruise. The mat itself doesn't need to be longer than the distance from the top of your head to the end of your tailbone.

In fair weather, toss a quilt on the lawn or beach.

Finding the Energy

There will be days when you don't want to work out. This is natural. Maybe it's raining. Your allergies are acting up. You're getting your period. However grumpy you feel, whatever mood you're in, whatever kind of day you're having, it's all irrelevant. You don't have to feel energetic. You don't have to feel any particular way. Just lie down, close your eyes, and open your mind.

Whatever else you're undergoing, all you have to do is commit yourself to your practice. Make a date with yourself, then simply lie down and follow through. Afterward, ask yourself if you're glad you did. Remember the paradox of exercise: As you expend energy, you create more of it. This is especially true of yoga.

Just trust you'll feel better once you get going. Sometimes students admit that they didn't want to practice because they were so exhausted. They wind up recharged. "After class I'm full of energy," remarks one, "and I like to jump up the stairs."

If you find yourself tired after yoga, this will pass. As you become more familiar with the work, you will be gaining both confidence and strength. Beneath the veneer of fatigue is pure energy. Eventually the natural state of well-being that you unearth can last for hours, even days. The effects are both immediate and cumulative.

A Note on Stretching

All stretches are rests. Ballistic bouncing is illegal here, as is any kind of forced motion. Your job is to surrender and let gravity do the work.

You must learn to distinguish between real pain and simple discomfort. Pain is always a cue to back off—to rest, breathe, and continue when and if you choose. Discomfort, on the other hand, is an invitation to linger longer and make yourself fully at home within the sensation.

In a way, it's like a party. You may feel uncomfortable in a new group of people, but if you use that discomfort as a ticket to linger instead of bolt, you may find yourself relaxing enough to enjoy yourself and even discover a friend. That's all we're doing, really—befriending the body and extending the borders of our comfort zone until we're at home in every position, anywhere we are. Sometimes muscles will quiver as you enter what we call the "trembling zone." Don't be afraid. You're changing.

In time the "path of breath" will extend naturally into the "path of stretch." The path of stretch is wherever in your body you feel the most happening at a given moment. It might be in the backs of your thighs on a forward bend, or the back of your waist on a spiral. With practice, once path breathing is well established, you can send the wind directly into what you are feeling, precisely where you feel it. The path of stretch is not unlike the path of a tornado or hurricane. Inside that whirlwind, in the center of the storm, is the eye of tranquillity. This is where you're heading in the midst of your sensations, as you follow your inner wind into the calm center of the stretch.

Finally, all stretches are multidirectional. That means we're moving in at least two directions, and sometimes three or more. If you feel lost, always refer to the core and extend the limbs from there.

Gentle Versions

Spread throughout the workout are Gentle Versions that modify the position or motion to suit various needs. If you're tired or achy or have specific physical issues, don't hesitate to use these modifications. In the course of a single workout, it's always up to you to decide how lightly or intensely to work your body. Listen well to what your body tells you.

Left Side First

To honor the neglected left side of the body, we always work the left side first in Yoganetics. In a society that has long emphasized right-side dominance in the physical arts, where manufacturers churn out right-handed gadgets, where four-way stops give the car on the right the right of way, where political fashion has even made "left" into a four-letter word, it is time to cheer for and strengthen the underdog. That means working the left side before the right, giving it the high priority of our first and finest attention. It is time to give the keys to the empty hand.

Standing Side Versus Moving Side

Sometimes we refer to one leg as the "standing leg." This term is imported directly from dance training and designates the leg that the dancer is standing on, as opposed to the "moving leg," which may be gesturing mid-air. Translated to Yoganetics, the standing leg is the one in direct contact with the floor while the moving leg is working in front, to the side, or behind the body. Likewise, the "standing arm" is the stabilizing arm pressing the floor. (Ditto "standing hand.")

The Class Structure

Yoganetics always begins with the voyage (chapter 3) and path breathing (chapter 4) to focus the attention within, anchor you to the core, and get the wind moving. Movement is then introduced as you continue to travel the path in reclining, sitting, and kneeling positions. Ultimately, all motions are woven into an hour-long movement meditation. We finish where we began, in Corpse Pose. In effect, all we've done is roll over, but you'll notice how very different the pose feels the second time around!

For a while you'll need to stop and start a bit while you acquaint yourself with each exercise. In time, when you've become familiar with the motions, you can practice using the Flow Chart at the end of the workout. It provides the sequence at a glance and includes page numbers for quick reference when you want to review instructions for a particular movement.

Each time you work out, read through the Ground Rules until they become bone deep—no, organ deep.

Ground Rules

1. Get in the Swim

Treat Yoganetics like a swimming class in two ways: Don't eat for at least an hour beforehand (two is better), and empty your bladder before beginning. The deep abdominal work we do makes a full stomach or bladder uncomfortable.

2. Say No to Strain and Pain

Never strain or force anything. This work is about getting to know your body on an intimate, organic level, and the first lesson is to listen when it tells you to let up. If something hurts, or if you feel dizzy or short of breath, stop and rest.

3. Drop the Form

You do not have to do everything in this workout. This cannot be overemphasized. Feel free to drop the *form* (the shape or motion) and simply practice the *content* (path breathing).

4. Be Beyond Compare

Compare yourself to no one—not to me, not to your friend, not even to yourself. You are an original. The purpose of this work is to become familiar with yourself, not to meet expectations (yours or anyone else's). Every time you do an exercise will feel different if you're paying attention, so don't confine your experience to what you've done before.

5. Feel Your Body

When you are asked to "feel" what's going on inside you, pay attention to your physical, visceral feelings, on the level of pure sensation. As muscles begin to release, emotions may also surface. This is a natural part of the process of reclaiming and transforming the body. Give yourself permission to let out and let go of whatever comes up.

6. Prefer the Left

As discussed, you will be working the left side of your body first, followed by the right side. The text always indicates in parentheses the direction of the first side—for instance, when you roll on your side (right first) to work the (left) leg. When you switch sides, simply reverse the direction in the parentheses.

7. Cluster Some Motions

A few of the exercises are clustered together. Occasionally, you are directed to proceed through all motions in the cluster before switching sides—for example, exercises 4 through 6.

8. Close Your Eyes

Yoganetics is done with the eyes closed to facilitate a deeper experience of the body as it moves. Feel free to cheat! Obviously, at first you will need to refer to the text. Open your eyes to read through the exercise. Then, as you grow comfortable, close them while you practice.

9. Exhale to Exert

In general, inhale to *prepare to move,* and exhale to *do the movement.* Inhale again on the return, and exhale to initiate or repeat the motion. The workout is designed so that you will be exhaling on the exertion, during the most challenging moments. Let the belly reflexively follow whatever the wind is doing.

10. Slow Down

Move in slow motion, as if underwater. Phrase the motion to the timing of the breath flowing through you, feeling every delicious sensation along the way. By slowing down, you'll notice when you're reaching the current boundary of your range of motion, which over time will naturally extend its borders.

Now turn off your phone, turn down the lights, and turn the page.

Six

Yoganetics for Beginners

If you put your ear to the ground now, you would hear the whole island seething with life.

J. M. BARRIE, *PETER PAN*

You may want to plunge right in, but before you begin the workout, do read the book up to this point. It will enable you to approach the work at a deeper level, enriching the experience of every move you make and every breath you take. Thus, you'll be using your time and energy more safely and effectively. If you have read the first five chapters, done the experiments, and practiced the voyage and path breathing, you are ready to embark.

Always review the Ground Rules (pp. 43–44) before you practice.

---

1. Corpse Pose

[for relaxation, realignment, rejuvenation]

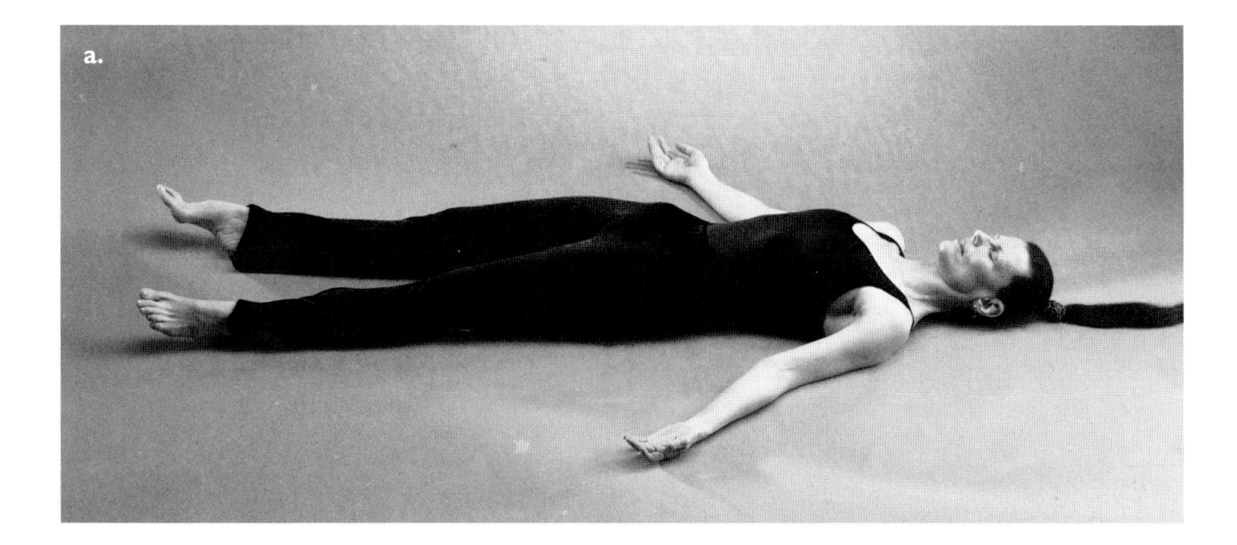

a. *The Voyage:* Lying on your back with legs and arms outstretched (legs hip-width apart, arms 45 degrees from your sides), turn the palms of the hands skyward. Drop the weight of the body into the earth. Close your eyes and take the voyage you've been practicing (pp. 22–26), mindfully moving from head to toe while releasing any tension you discover. [5 *minutes*]

Gentle Version: *Bend your knees and plant your feet on the floor hip-width apart.*

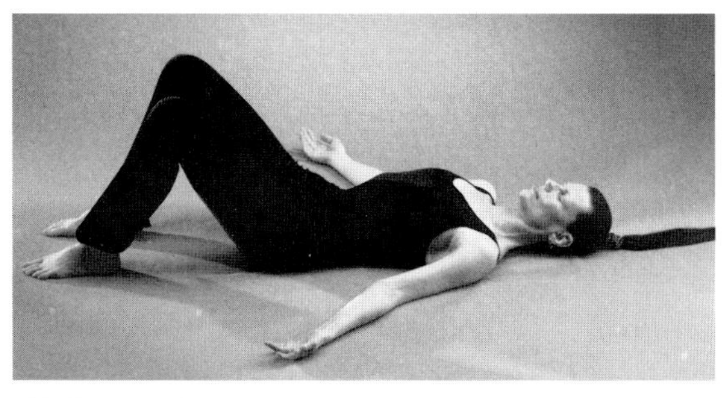

GENTLE VERSION

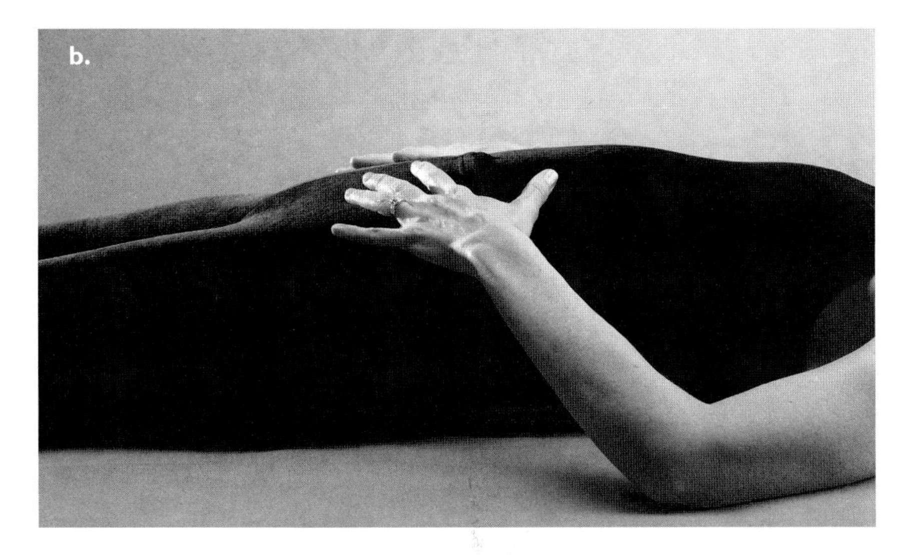

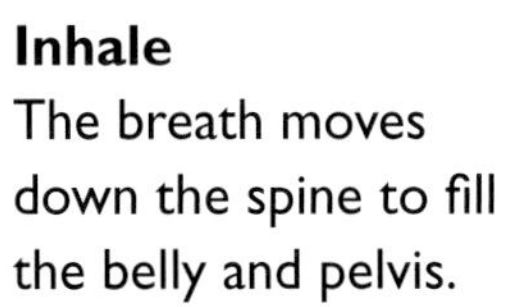

Inhale
The breath moves down the spine to fill the belly and pelvis.

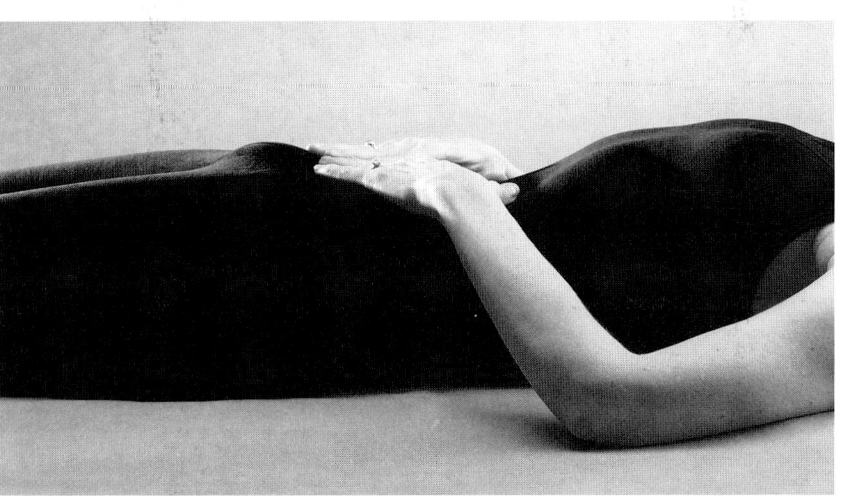

Exhale
The breath moves up the spine, the belly falling and following through.

b. *The Path [for lungs, abdominals, reintegration]:* Place your hands on your low belly between the hipbones. Bring your attention up inside the heart center. Inhale as you feel the wind moving downward to fill the belly. Exhale and let the belly fall, following the breath inward to the spine and upward through the heart. Keep traveling the path of breath between the heart and gravitational center as you inhale and exhale. [*8 slow breaths*]

2. Tail Curls

[for abdominals, inner thighs, hamstrings, spine]

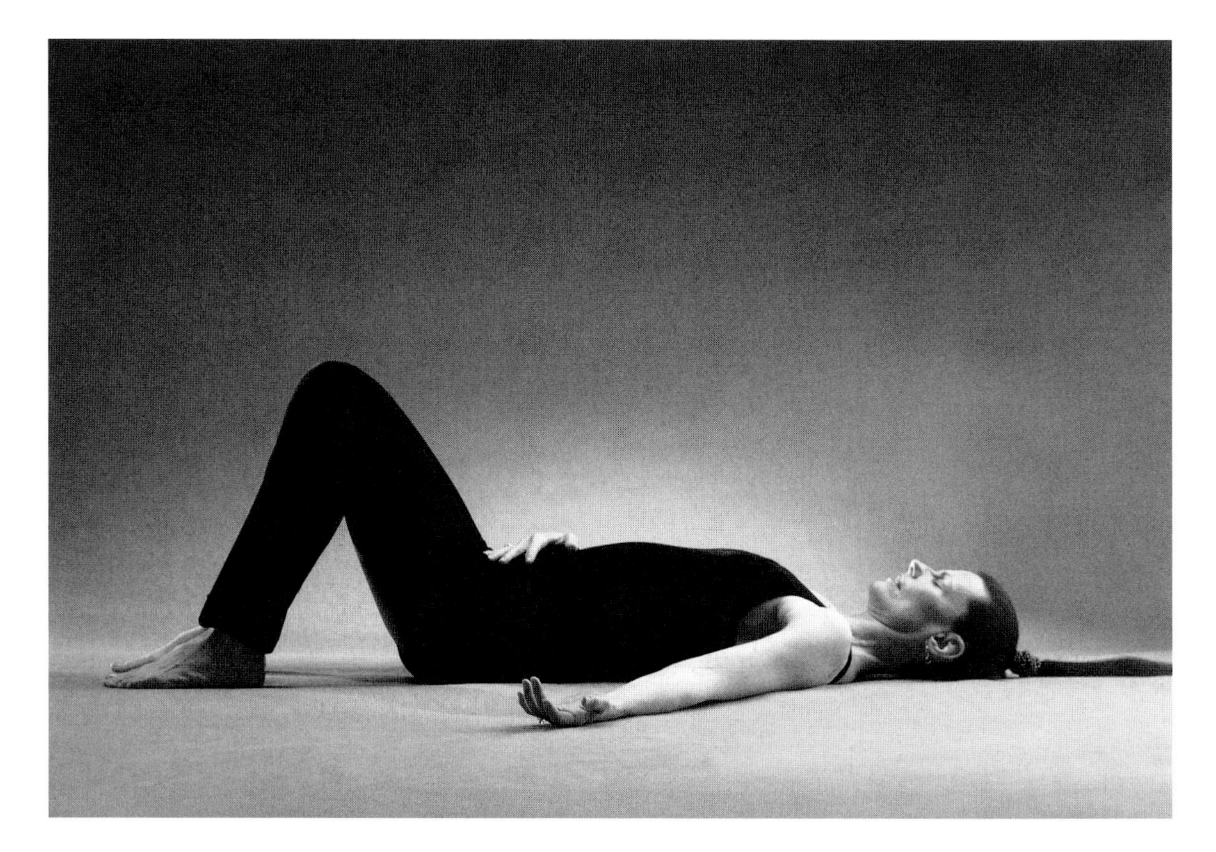

PREPARATION

Bend your knees and plant the feet hip-width apart on the floor, toes in line with heels. Inhale, feeling the wind move below the belt to fill the cave of your belly.

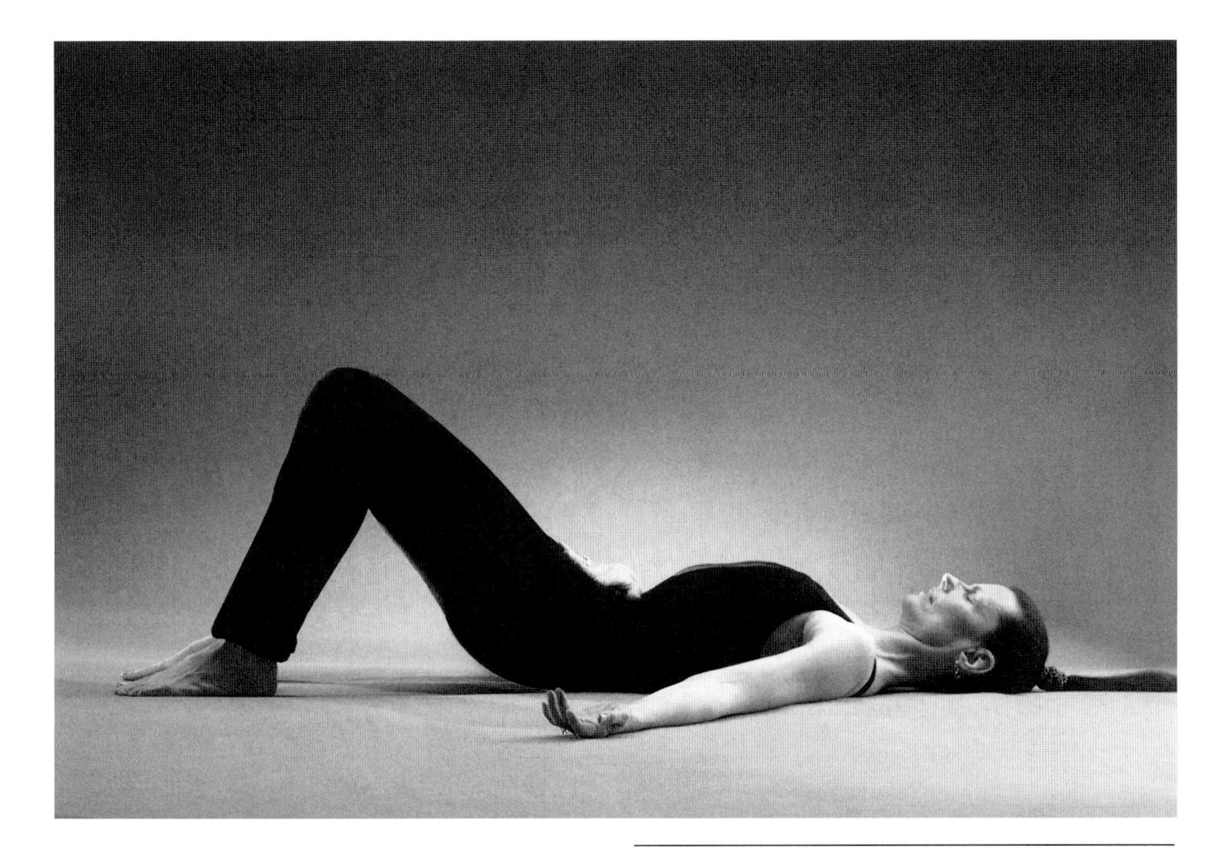

MOTION

Exhale, spreading the toes and pressing your feet into the earth as you curl your tailbone slightly up toward the sky, feeling the belly collapse on exhalation. Inhale, filling the cave again as your tail unrolls to earth. [*8 times*]

Tip: *The back of the waist stays on the floor throughout. Are you favoring the gas pedal foot? During each Tail Curl, push the feet down and the crown of the head up, out of the core.*

3. Double Leg Press

[for spine, digestion, circulation]

PREPARATION

Fold knees to chest and wrap your arms around the backs of your thighs, legs hip-width apart. Pressing the legs comfortably close to the body, drop your chin and lengthen the back of the neck. Notice the lower back spreading open. Inhale, breathing downward into the belly, pelvis, and seat.

MOTION

Exhale, following the underflow of wind along the spine. Your legs will fall naturally closer to the body as the belly gets out of the way. [*4 breaths*]

Tip: *The lower back and hips stay on the floor. Relax your shoulders throughout.*

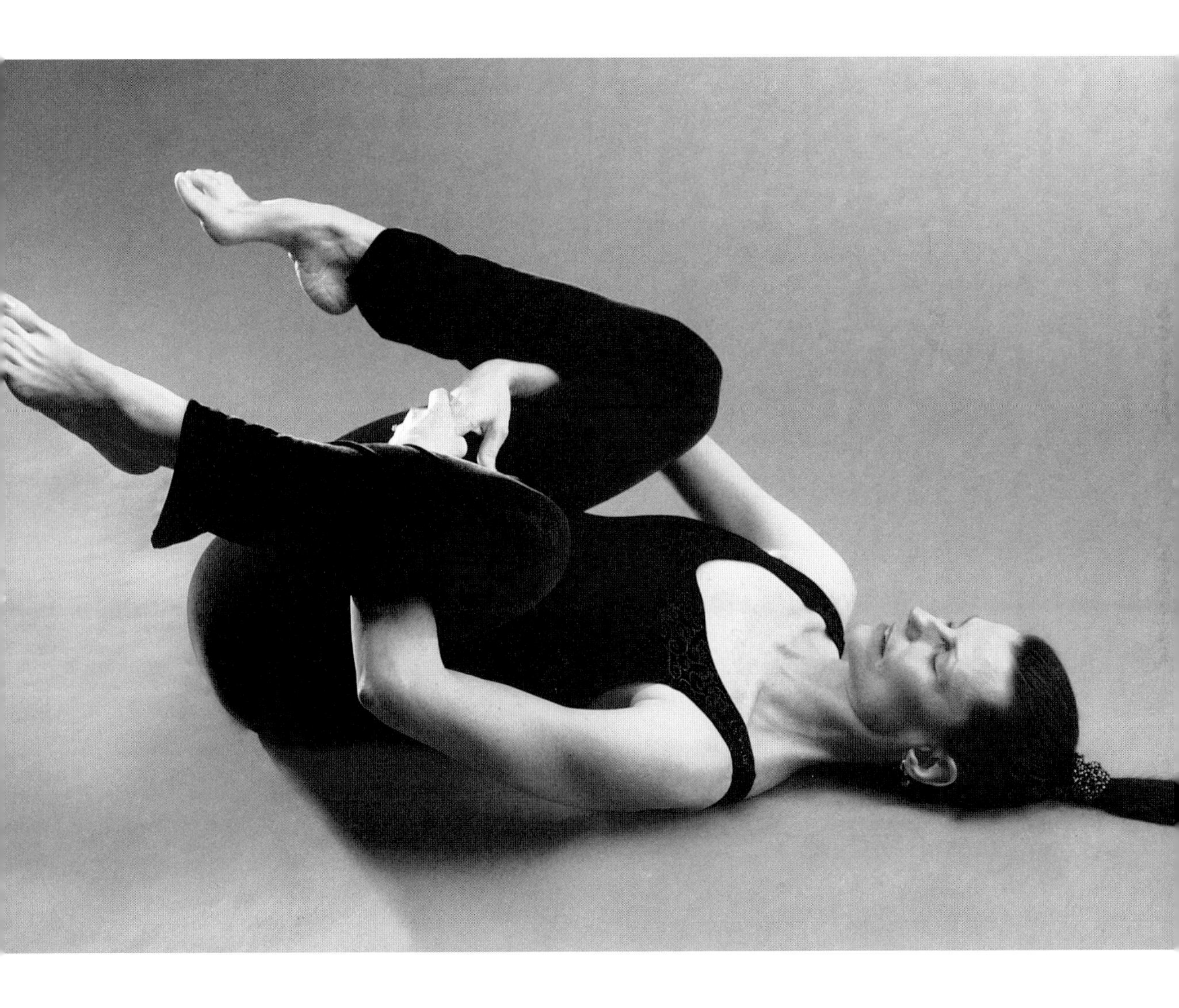

4. Thigh Circles

[for opening hip joint]

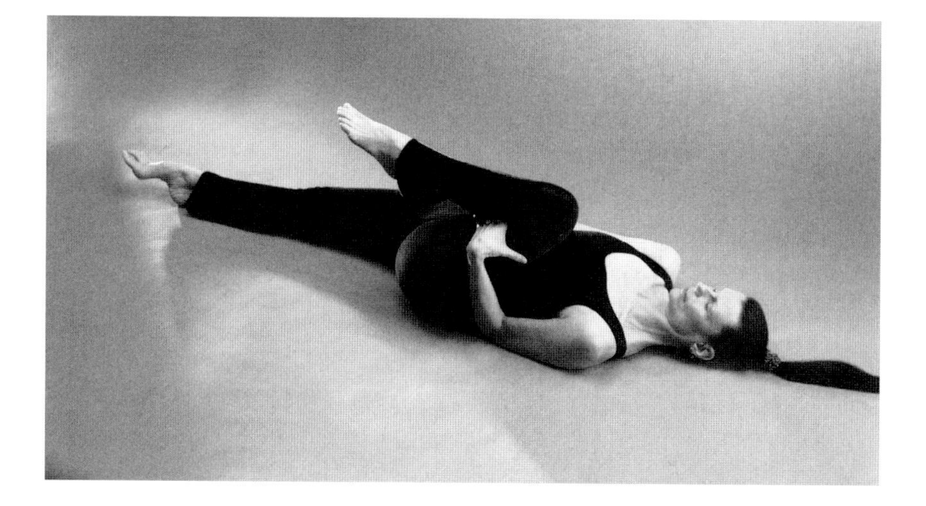

PREPARATION

Bend your knee (left first) and hold the thigh, extending the other leg along the floor.

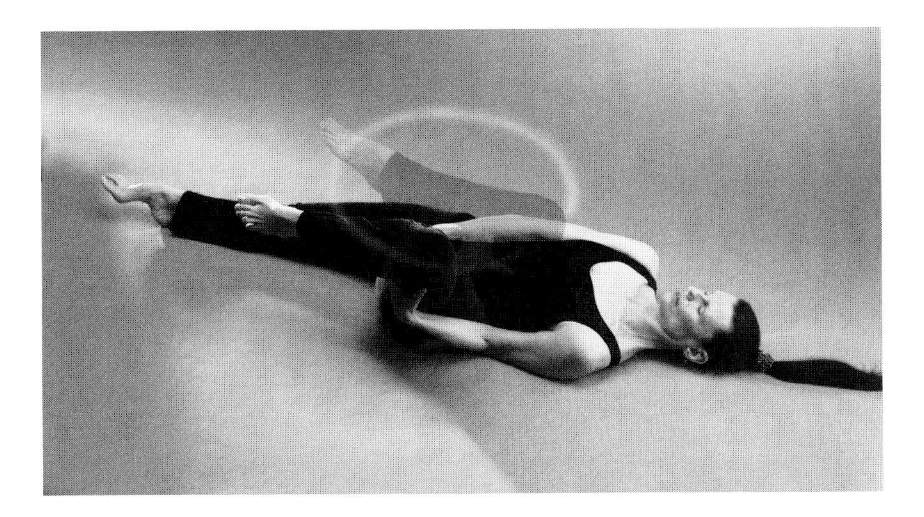

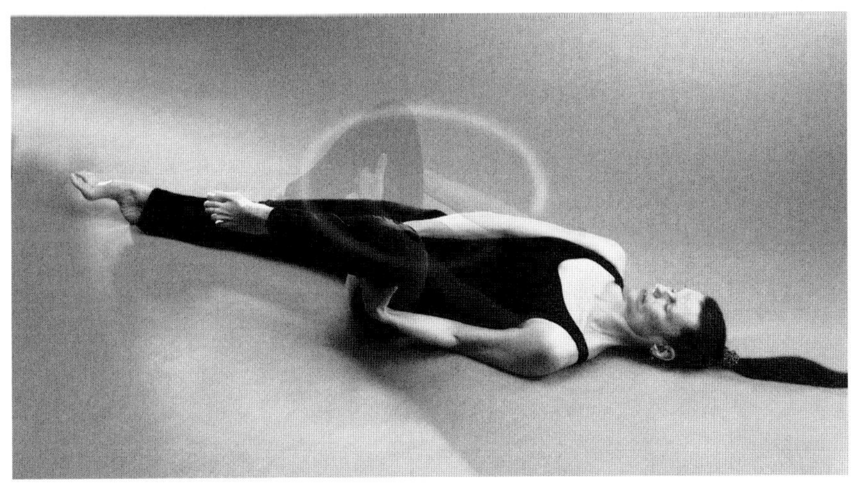

MOTION

Using the arms to guide your femur, slowly draw big circles with your knee, moving it like the second hand of a clock. [*4 times, then reverse direction. Proceed through exercises 5 and 6 before switching sides.*]

***Tip:** Relax the shoulders throughout. If any numbers on your clock's circle are difficult for you, linger and breathe into them.*

5. Separated Leg Push

[for hamstrings, quadriceps, calves, inner thighs, spine]

PREPARATION

Still holding your thigh (the other leg long along the earth), inhale, filling the belly.

MOTION

Exhale, flexing your feet and extending both legs as straight as possible, pushing your top heel into the sky. Feel the belly fall as the wind flows upward through the heart, pushing both heels equally and endlessly out of the cave and into the world. Inhale and return, bending your top knee. [*4 times. Also do exercise 6 before switching sides.*]

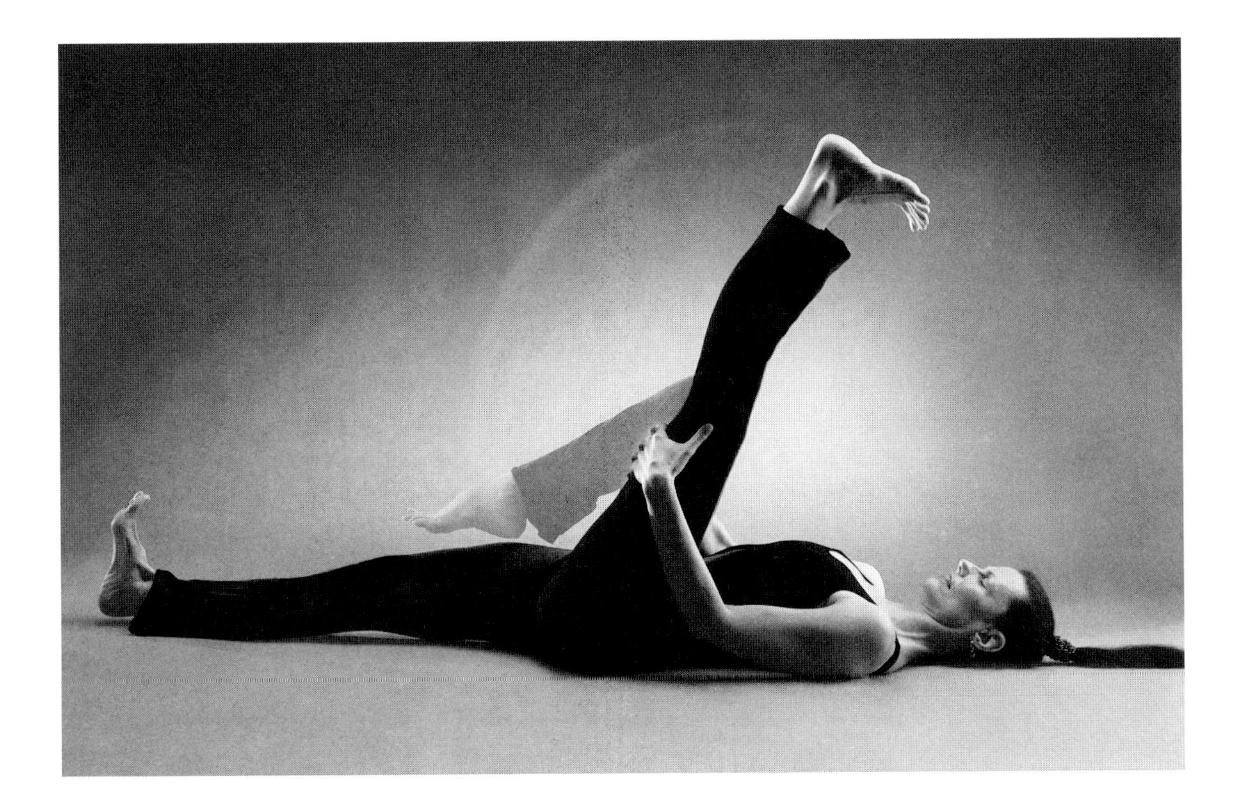

Tip: *Don't be concerned if your top leg doesn't straighten. It's far more important to push the heel of the leg on the floor—as well as the crown of the head—out of the cave, elongating the entire body.*

GENTLE VERSION

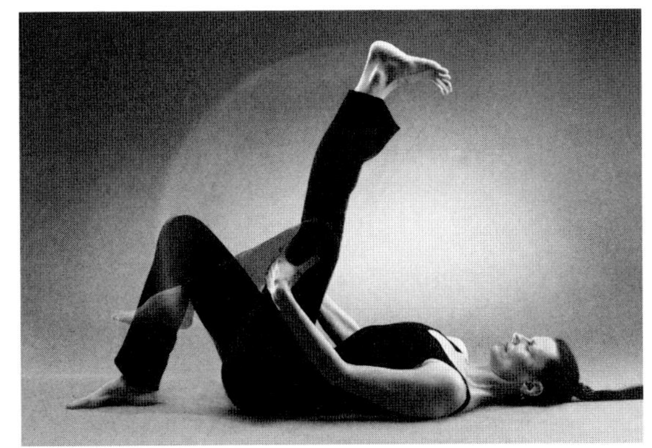

Gentle Version: *Bend the standing leg and plant the foot on the floor, keeping this leg bent throughout.*

6. Supported Single Legovers

[for opening spine, heart]

PREPARATION

Plant the foot of the leg you've just been working on the floor beside the knee of the extended leg. With your opposite hand, take the knee across the body, letting the hip come off the floor and resting the foot on the inside of the standing leg. Lengthen your other arm in the opposite direction, palm facing the sky. Anchor both shoulders on the floor. Inhale and relax, breathing into the stretch behind the waist.

MOTION

Exhale, looking back over the shoulder of your outstretched arm, lengthening the arm along the earth and pushing through your fingertips. [*3 breaths. When finished, change sides and repeat 4, 5, and 6 with the right leg.*]

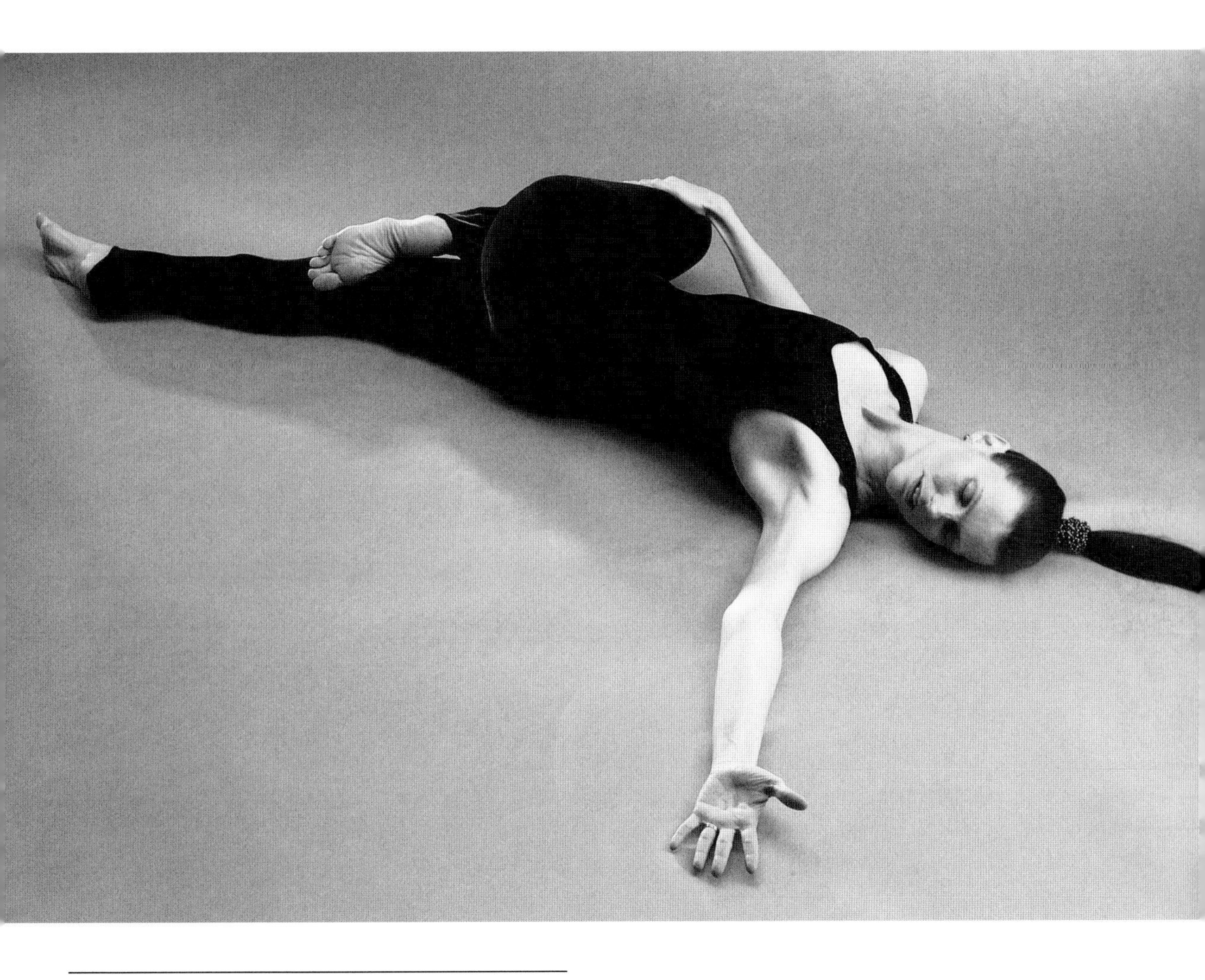

***Tip:** The shoulder of the extended arm stays grounded throughout.*

7. Groaner

[for outer thighs, buttocks]

PREPARATION

Rolling onto your side (right first), rest your head on your arm and bend the knees 90 degrees at hip level, shins parallel to spine. Line up the top shoulder directly over your bottom shoulder, top hip directly over bottom hip. The free arm rests in front of your body, palm up. Inhale, filling the cave.

MOTION

a. Exhale, lifting the top leg (left first) about 10 inches. Inhale, lowering the leg *almost* all the way. [*4 to 8 times slow, then 16 pulses, exhaling with each pulse*]

b. Extend your top leg forward, foot parallel to the floor. Exhale, slowly lifting the leg without moving the top hip. Inhale, lowering the leg back to hip height. [*4 to 8 times slow, 16 pulses. Before switching sides, do exercise 8 as a counterpose.*]

MIRROR IMAGE

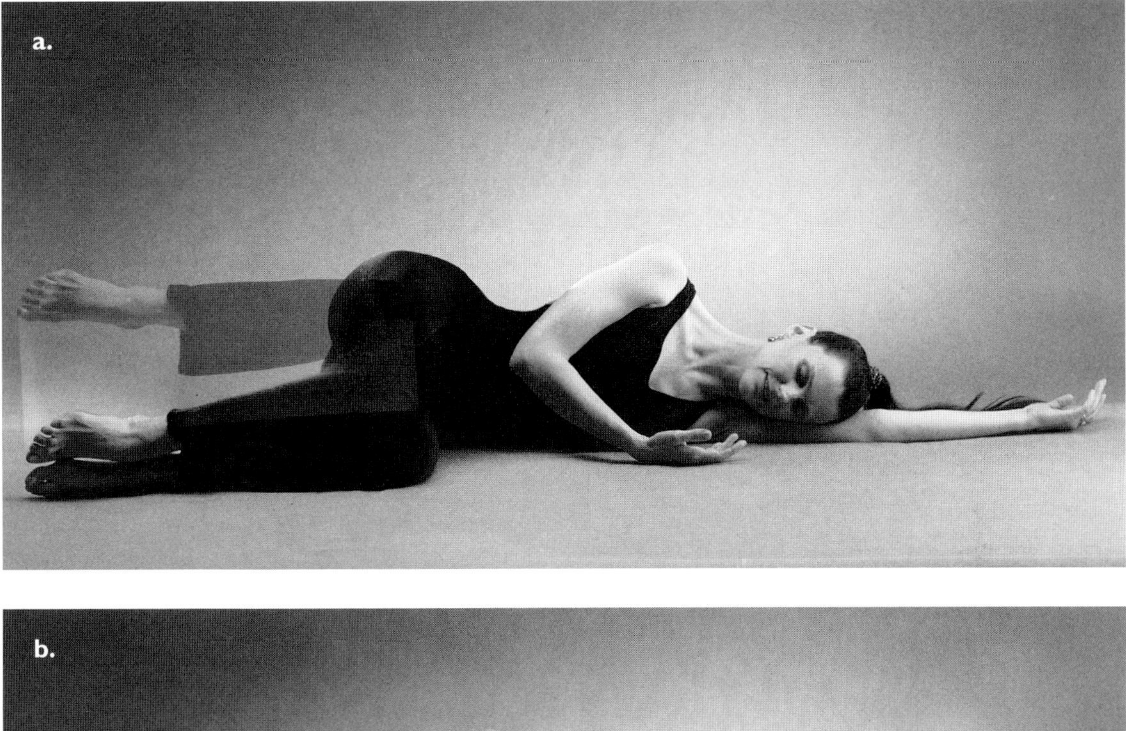

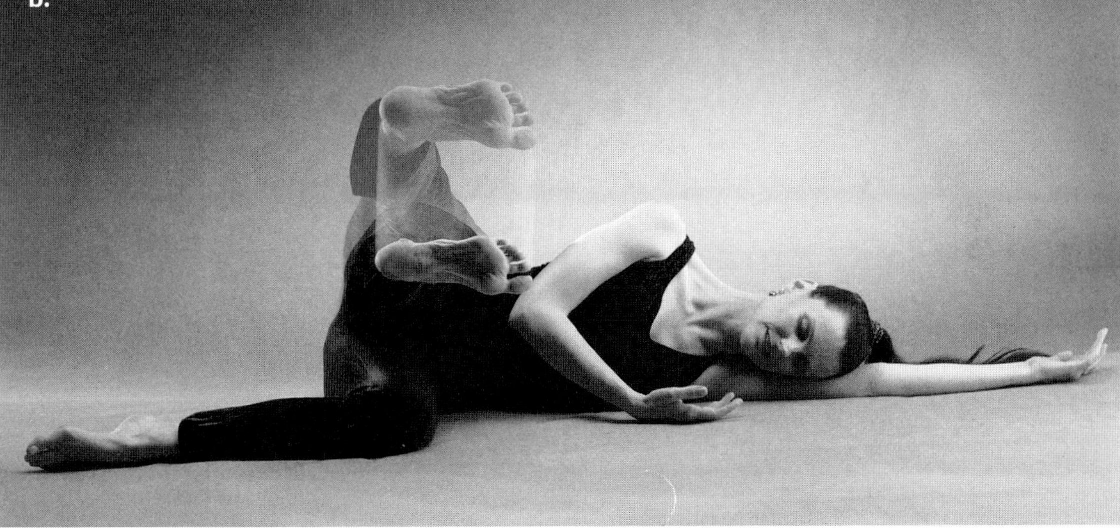

Tip: *Don't let the top hip fall back as you lift your leg. Maintain your alignment (shoulder over shoulder, hip over hip) throughout. Your goal is to drop deep within and follow the path of wind.*

8. Barn Door

[for hips, buttocks]

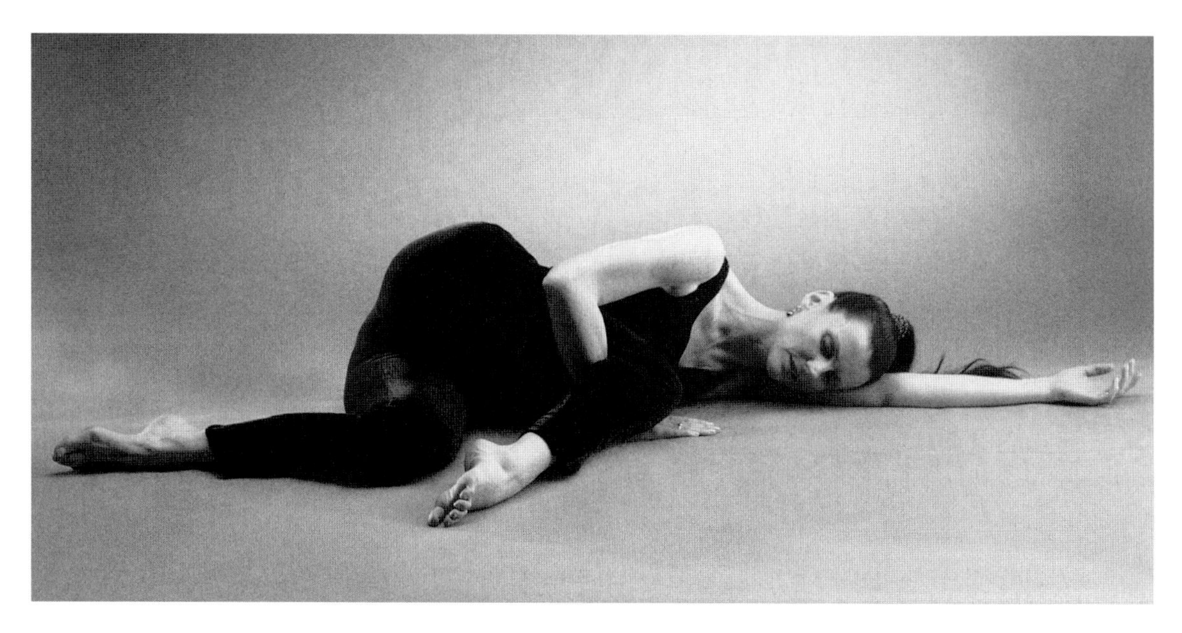

PREPARATION

Staying on your side, bring the thigh (left first) to your chest and rest.

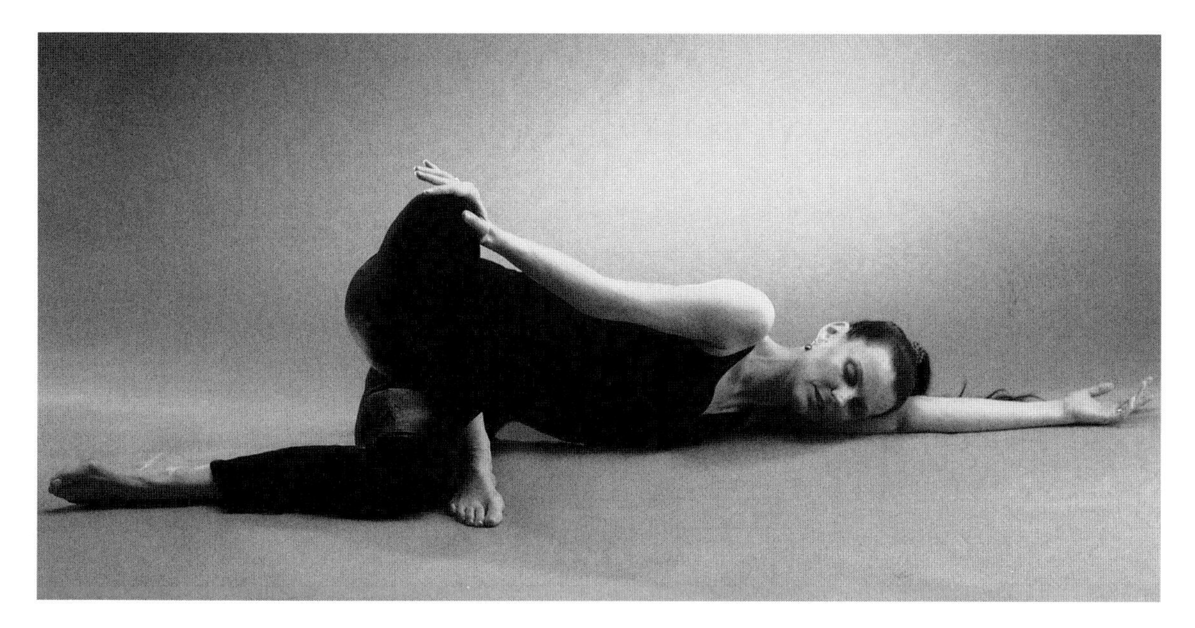

MOTION

Plant the foot of the leg you just worked on the floor above the other knee. Press your top knee open with your top hand. Inhale and breathe directly into the area you feel the most, letting light and wind into the hay-filled barn of the buttock, where all the animals are sleeping.

Exhale and gently press the knee open like a barn door. Inhale and repeat. [*3 breaths, then switch sides and repeat exercises 7 and 8*]

9. Easy Flatback

[for hips, spine]

PREPARATION

Using your arms, walk yourself up to a sit, then fold your legs together. Inhale, sitting tall and filling the belly.

MOTION

a. Exhale and move forward, keeping your spine straight and the front of your torso long. Place the hands in front of you on the floor and relax. Inhale, filling the belly, hips, lower back, and wherever else you may feel this stretch. Exhale and lengthen the spine, moving your lower back closer to the legs if comfortable, without rounding the spine. *[4 breaths]*

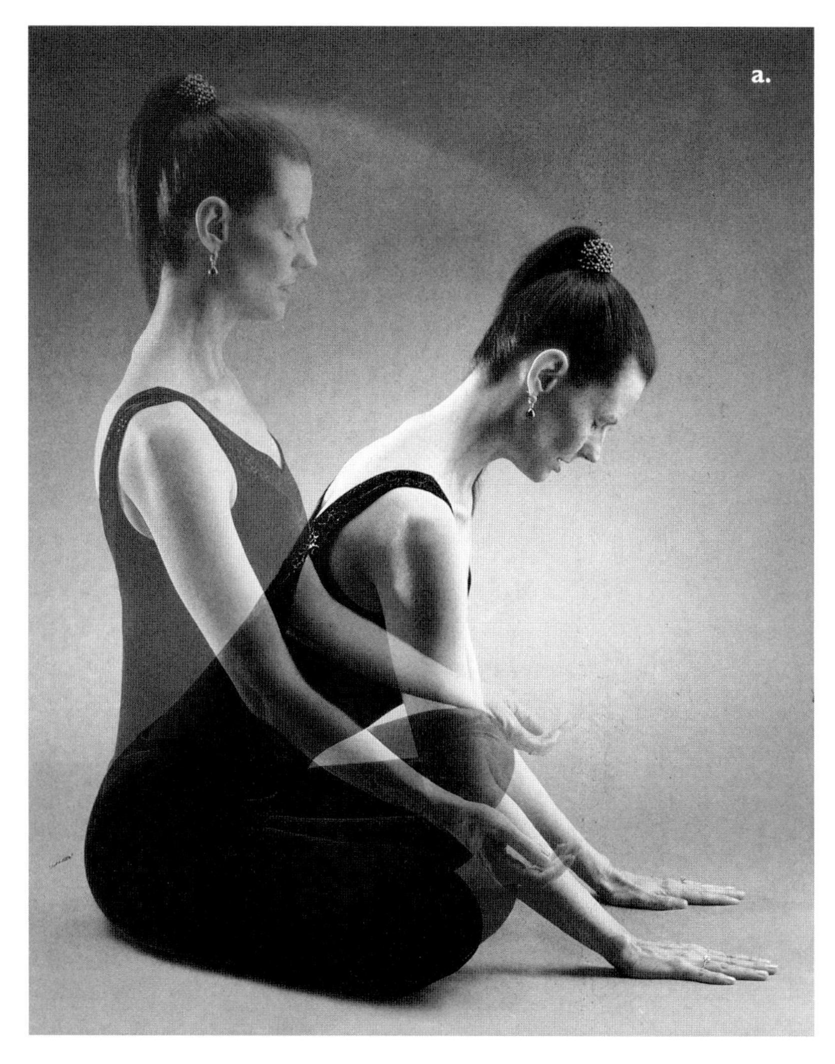

Gentle Version:
If sitting with a straight back is difficult, fold or roll up your mat or towel and place it under your hips.

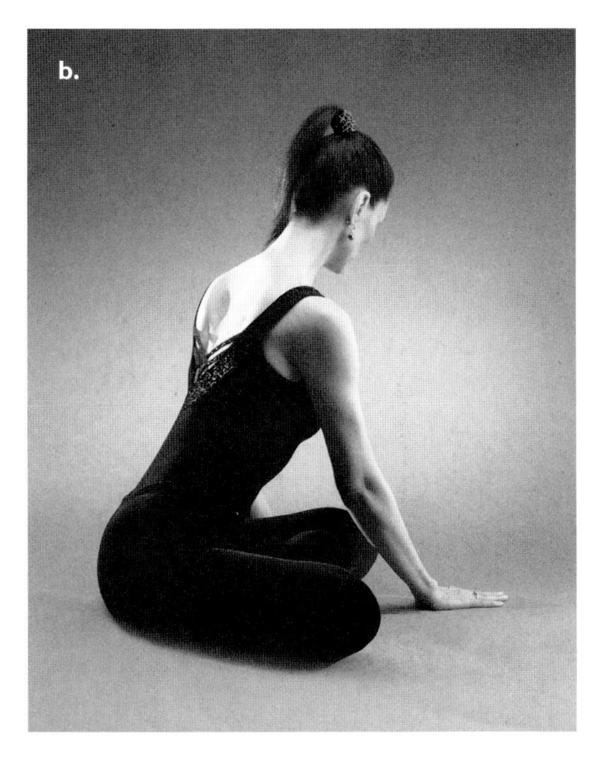

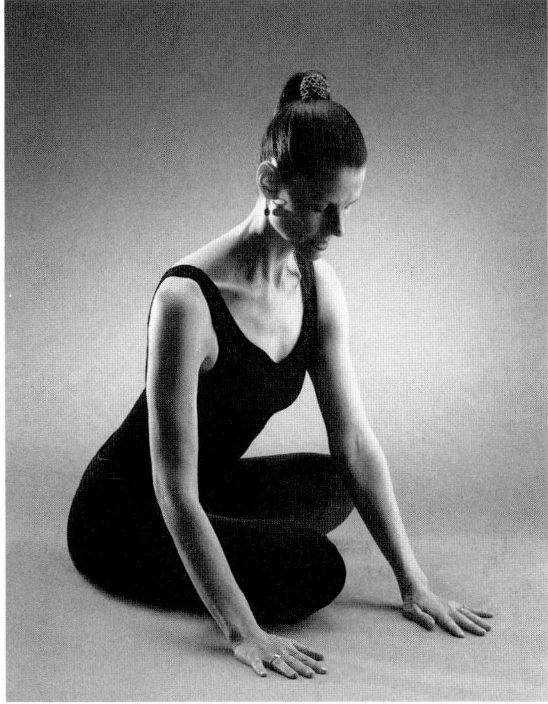

b. Inhale and turn toward your (left) leg. Exhale and move out over the leg, keeping the back flat and the opposite hip weighted. Inhale and fill the stretch; exhale and let yourself lengthen and deepen into this pose. [*2 breaths. Repeat on the right side.*]

Tip: *Bend from the hips, not the waist. When you move over one leg, keep the opposite hip on the floor.*

10. Folding Tree

[for spine, backs of legs]

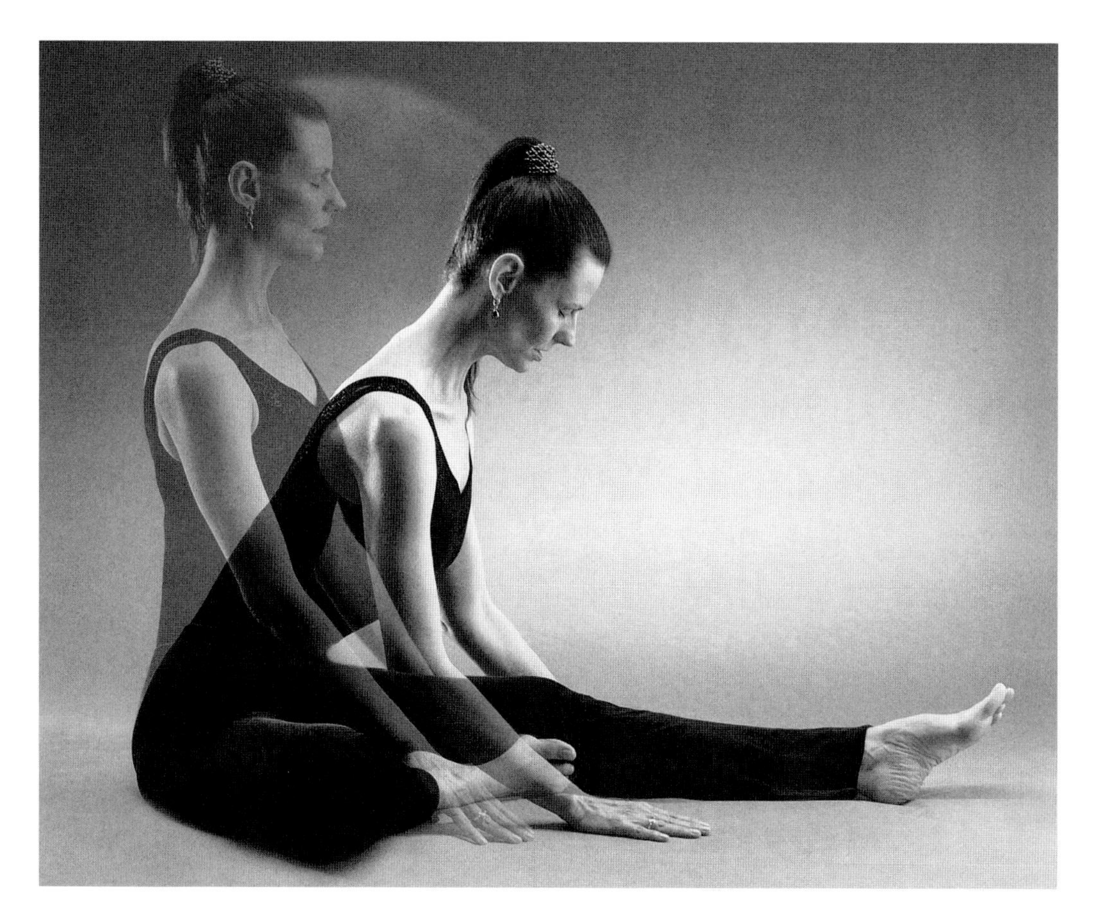

Still sitting, extend the (left) leg in front of the hip. Open the other knee outward and place the foot beside the extended thigh. With a flat back, bend forward from the hips, your hands straddling the extended leg. Linger here and breathe into the path of stretch as and where you experience it. [*3 breaths. Proceed through exercise 11 before changing legs.*]

Tip: *Bend from the hips, not the waist, keeping the spine straight all the way through the back of the neck and pointing the crown of the head like a magician's hat. You may not bend very far forward here, but a flat back is crucial, even if the extended leg has to bend a bit.*

GENTLE VERSION

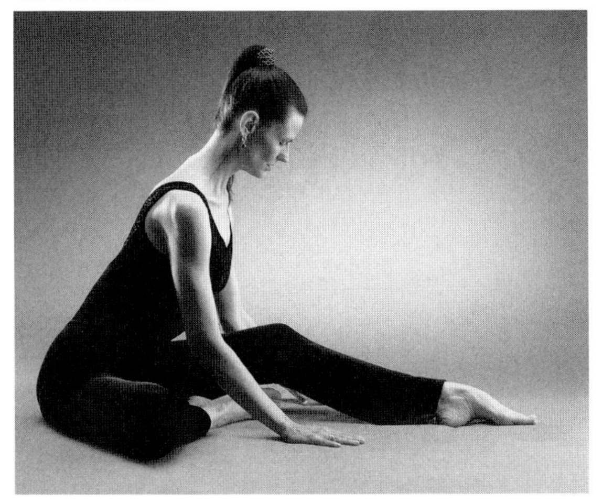

Gentle Version: *Bend the extended leg slightly for your flatback stretches.*

CHALLENGE VERSION

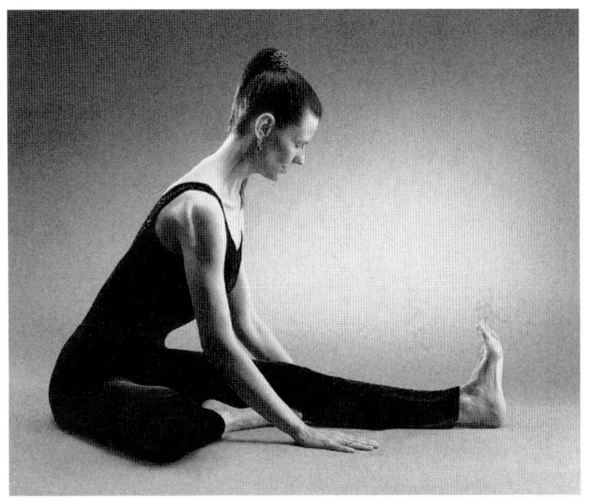

Challenge Version: *If your spine is straight and your leg is straight, you can intensify the stretch by flexing the foot and pushing out through the heel.*

11. Tree Spiral

[for spine, organs, hips]

PREPARATION

With your leg still extended and the other knee still bent, hop the foot of the bent leg over the extended knee and plant the foot on the floor. Turn toward your bent leg and embrace it with your opposite arm. The other hand (right first) is planted on the floor behind you, the heel of the hand toward the body. Inhale, filling the belly.

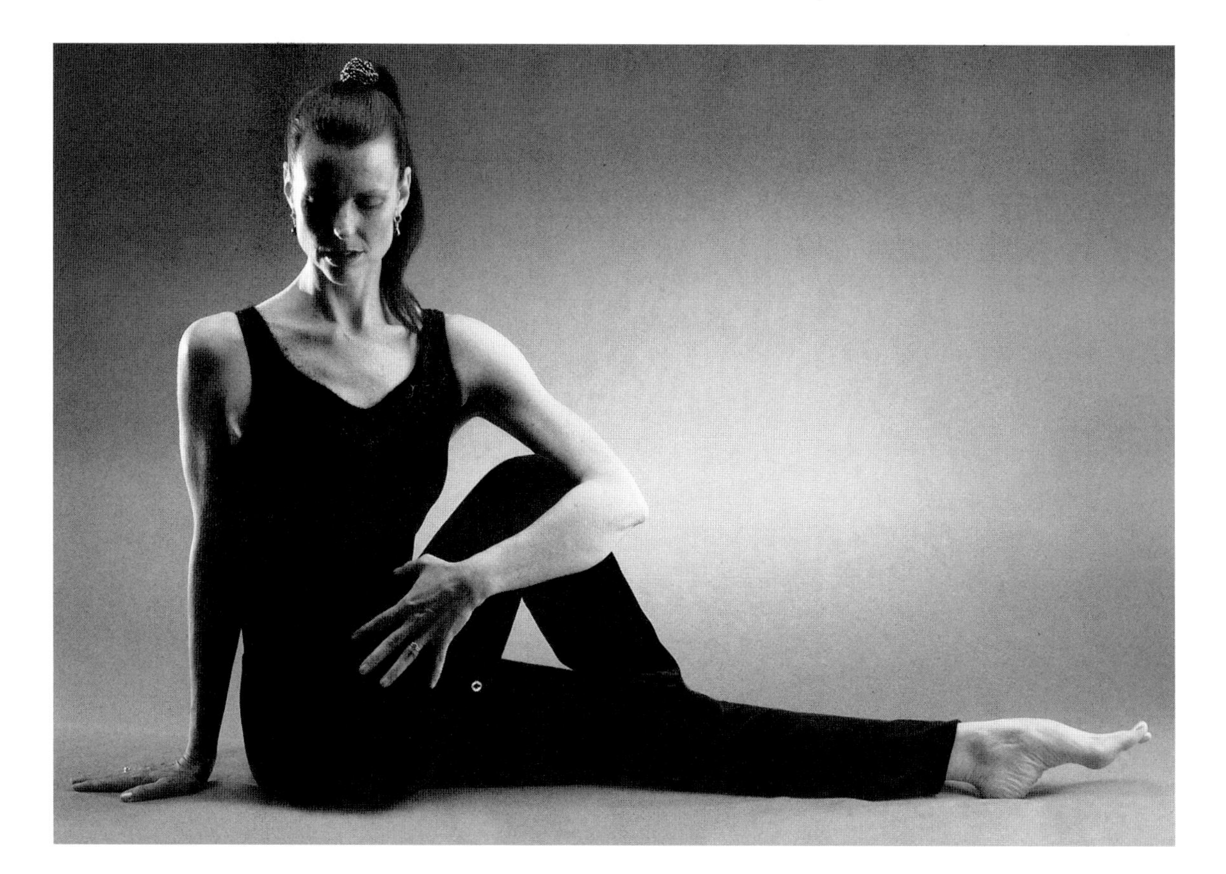

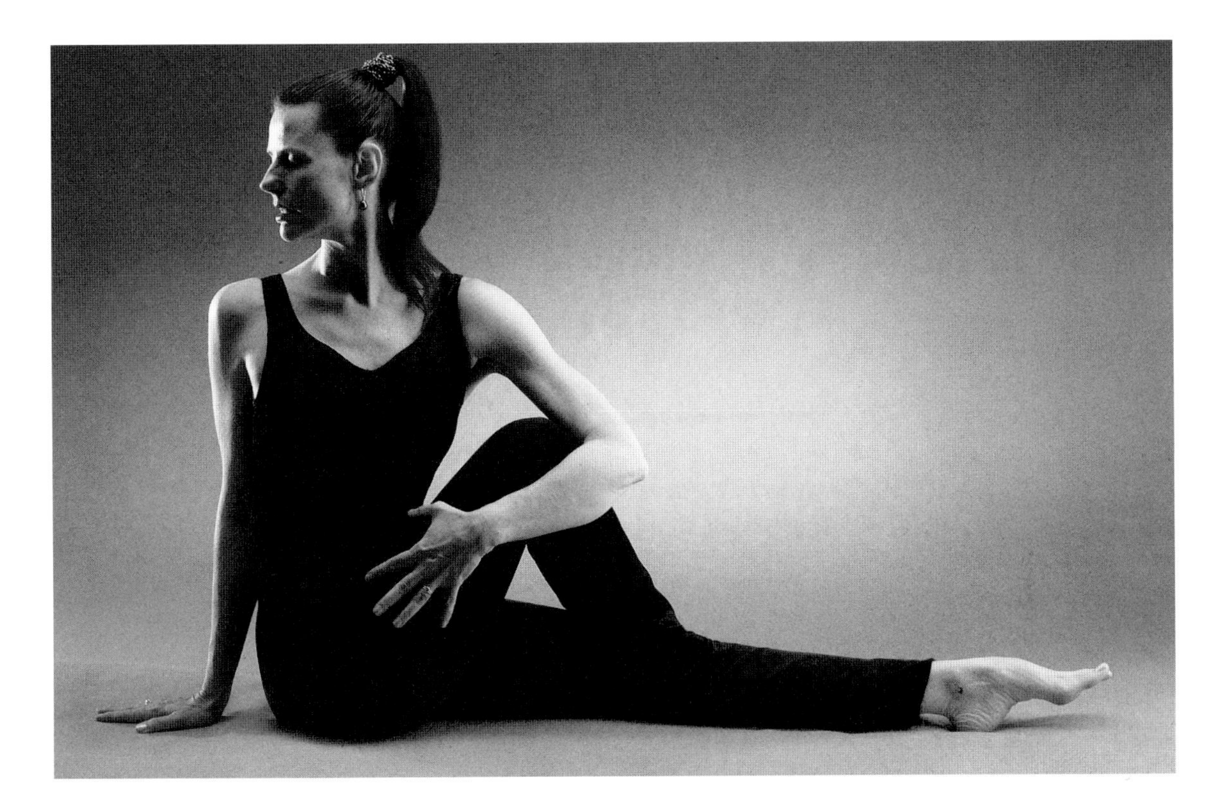

MOTION

Exhale, pressing the thigh close, turning your body toward the bent leg, and looking beyond the back shoulder. Inhale, unwinding enough to fill the belly, then exhale and turn a little further. [*3 breaths. Switch sides and repeat exercises 10 and 11 before going further.*]

Tip: *Push the crown of your head up out of the belly and stay tall throughout. Don't over-rely on the arms; spiral from the core outward.*

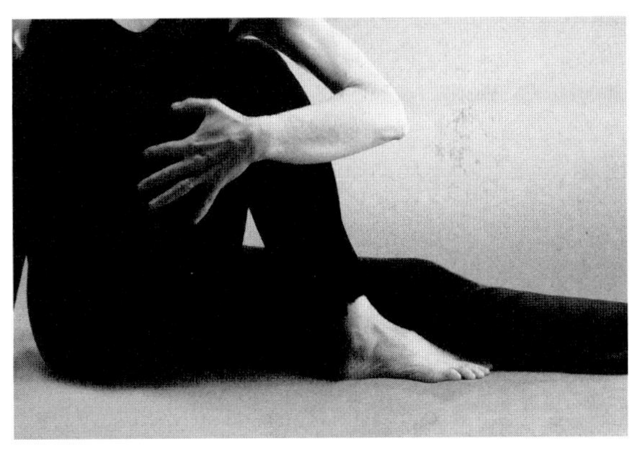

GENTLE VERSION

Gentle Version: *Don't hop over the extended leg with your foot. Instead, plant your foot on the floor just inside the extended leg.*

---

12. Rear Window

[for lower back]

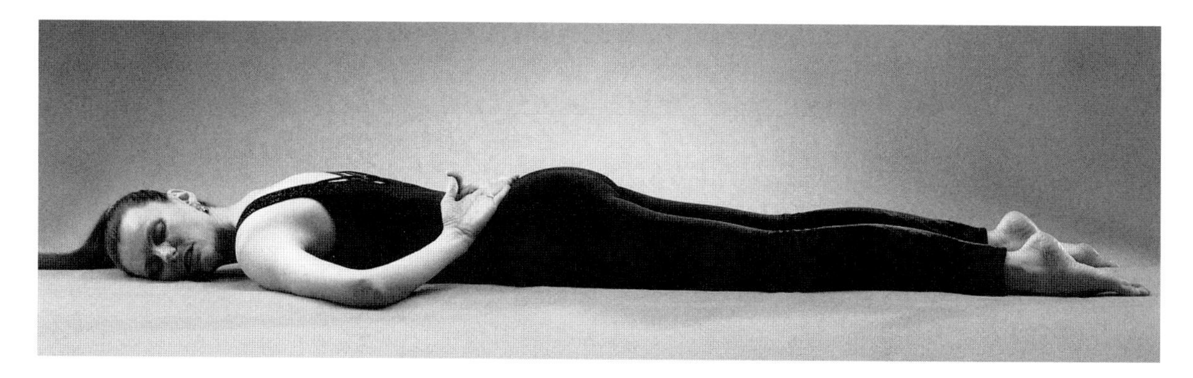

Lie down on your belly and let your legs sprawl. Rest your hands on your lower back below the waist. Close your eyes and visualize the lower back as an open window. Starting from the heart center, inhale directly into the hands, through the secret window. The back will rise, like silk curtains lifted by wind. Now exhale, feeling the lower back drift down as the curtains fall back to the sill. [*4 breaths*]

Gentle Version: *If your back doesn't like this position, roll up your mat or towel and place it under your belly. If your hands aren't happy on the lower back, fold them under your brow or place them at your sides.*

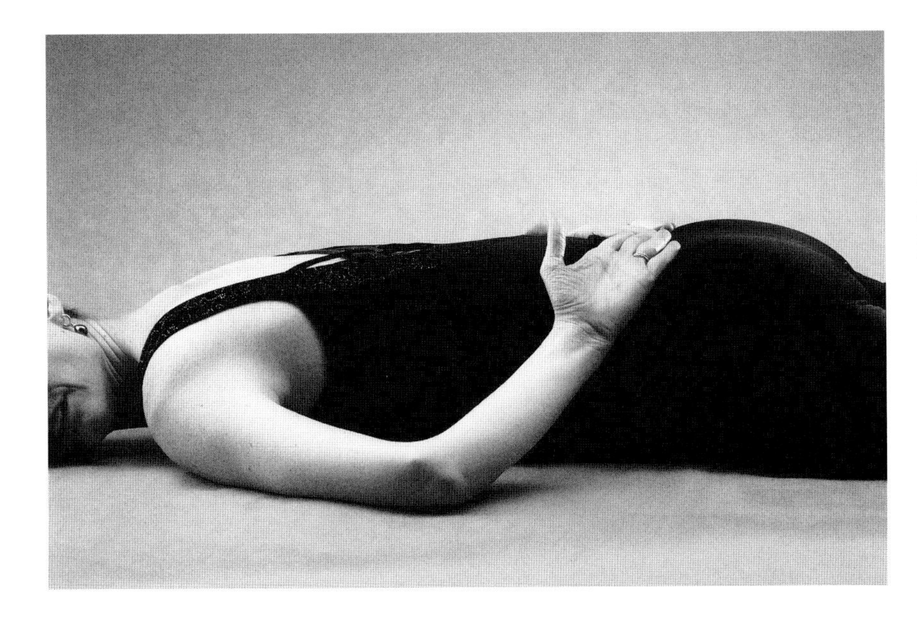

Inhale
Feel the lower back rise.

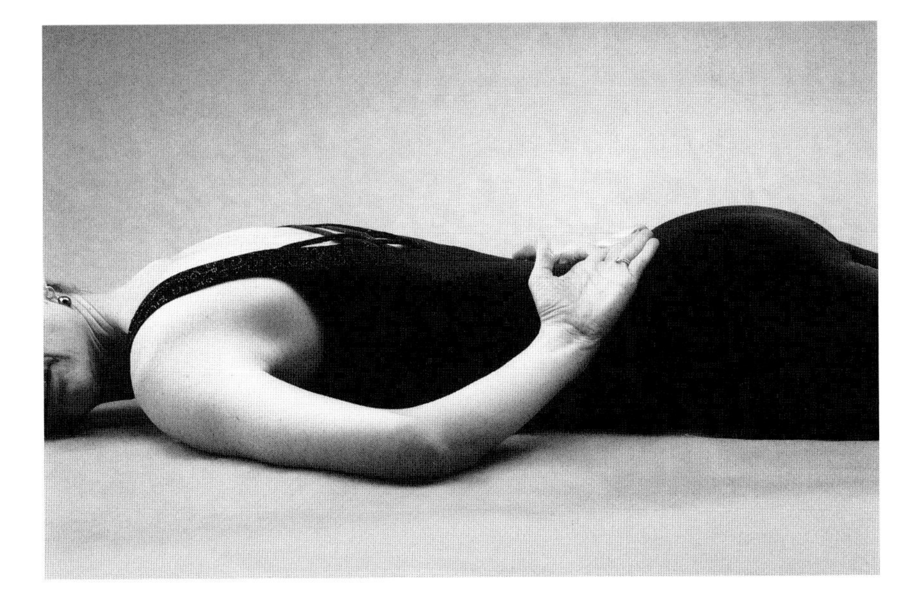

Exhale
Feel the lower back drift down.

13. Pre-Cobra

[for core abdominal muscles, spine]

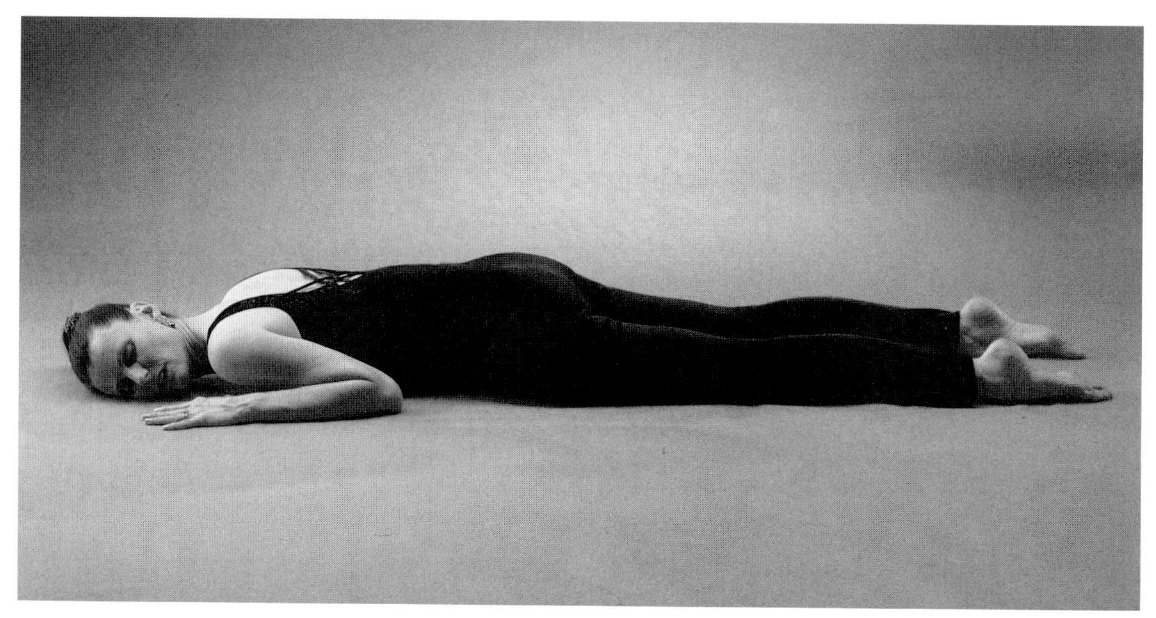

PREPARATION

Still prone, place your hands beneath your shoulders, palms down, fingers spread, elbows on the floor beside the ribs. Inhale and fill the lower back.

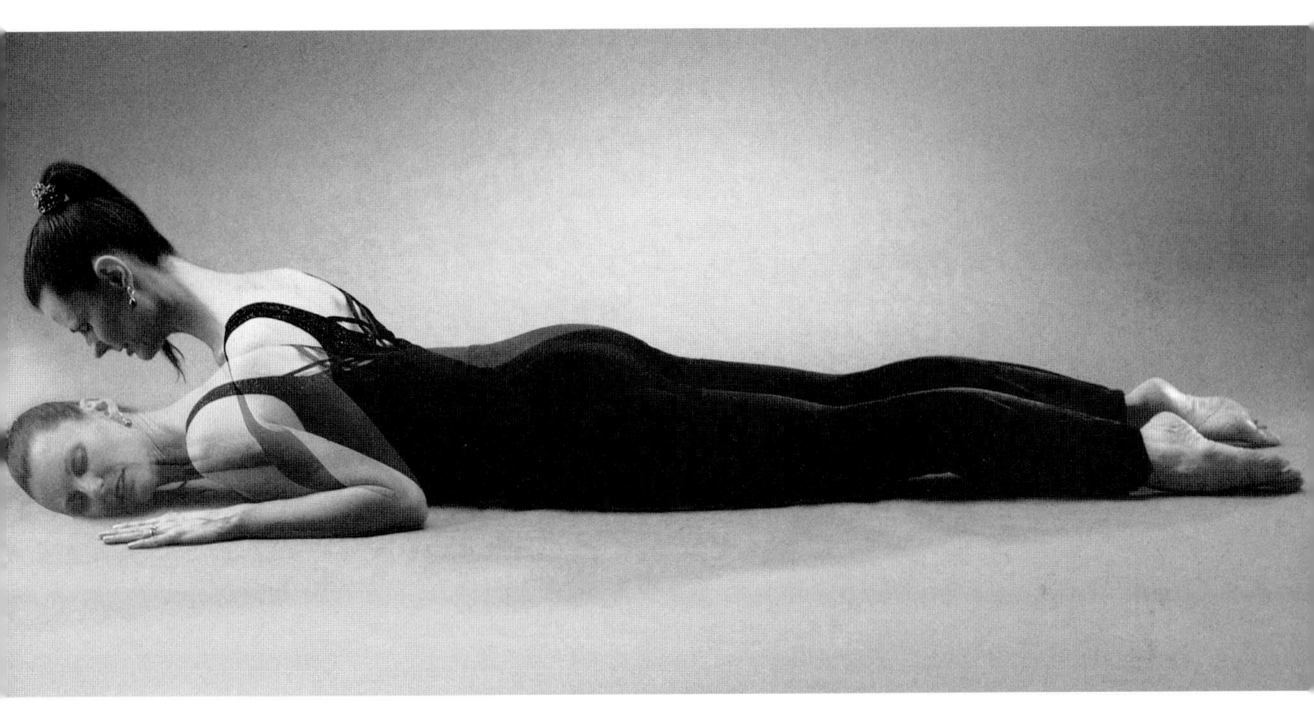

MOTION

Exhale, first elongating the spine through the crown of the head, then lifting the upper body off the floor as far as you can without using the arms. Inhale and gently lower, filling the lumbar chamber. [*4 times*]

Tip: *When lifting your head, tilt the chin in, push the crown out, and don't break the line of the neck. Although the low-back muscles are working here, go deeper to the core and source the motion in the abdominal cave.*

14. Lateral Cat

[for waist, spine]

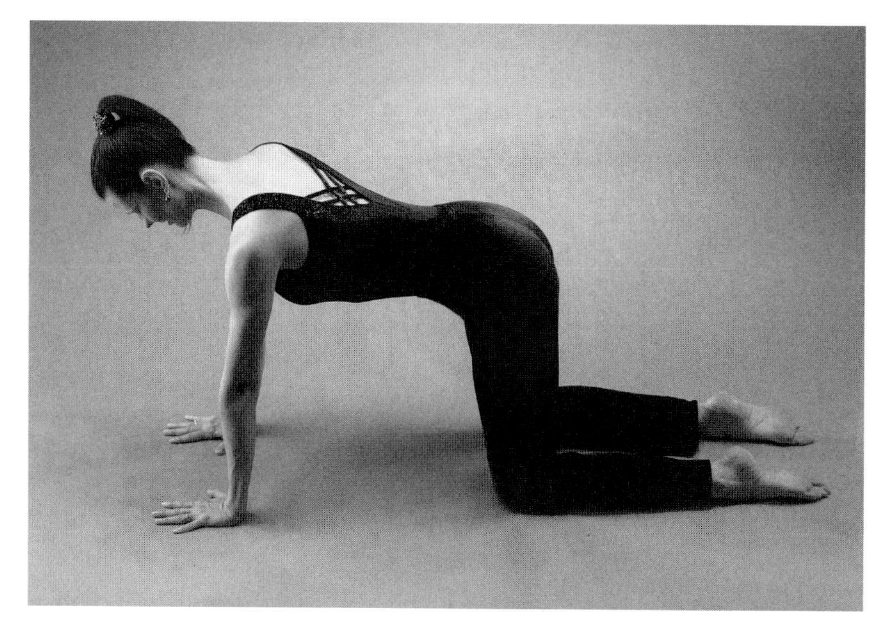

PREPARATION

Pushing up to your hands and knees, place your hands directly beneath your shoulders, knees beneath hips, hip-width apart. The back is flat, head in line with spine. Inhale, filling the belly.

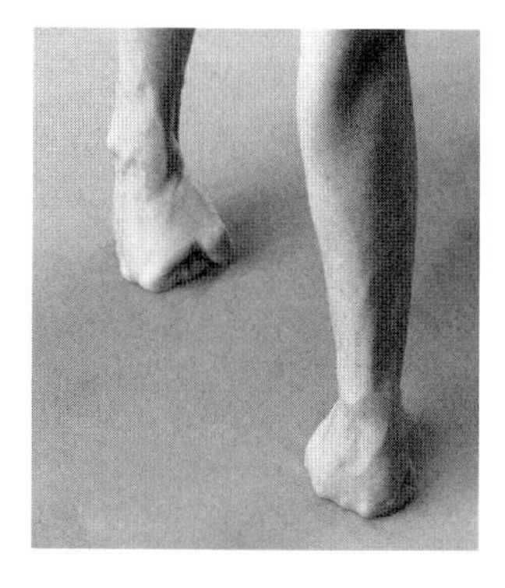

Gentle Version: *If this hurts your wrists, rise up on your fists.*

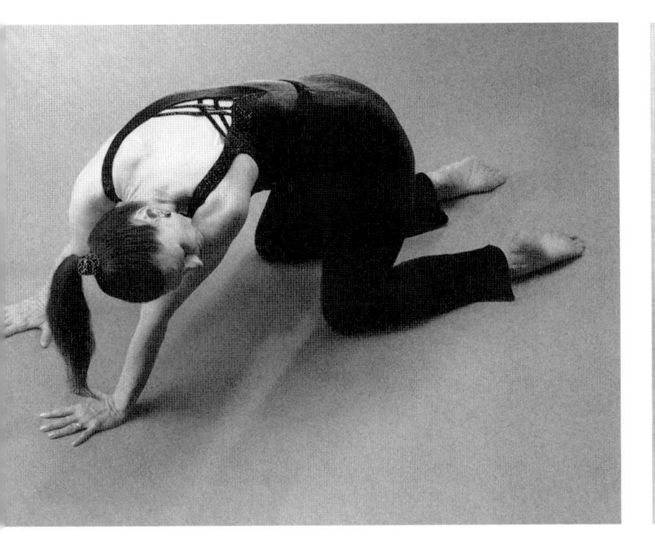

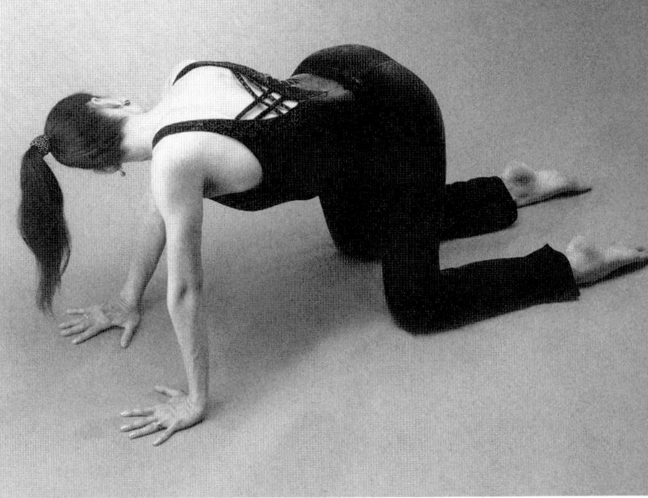

MOTION

Exhale, turning both your head and hips to the side (left first), the head and tail looking for each other as if trying to meet. Feel the opposite side-seam stretching its stitches. Inhale and fill the path of the stretch, then exhale and twist a little further. Inhale and return to center. Exhale and turn the other way. [*4 times, alternating left and right*]

Tip: *Keep the arms actively straight throughout, pushing the earth away.*

15. Cat

[for spine, inner thighs, abdominals, hamstrings]

PREPARATION

Still on your hands and knees, point and spread the fingers forward, actively pushing through the arms. Lift the head and tail and inhale, letting the belly drop downward.

MOTION

Exhale and find your tailbone, pulling it down toward the earth. Roll through the lower back, middle back, and upper back until the head finally drops and the back of your heart pushes skyward. Inhale and unroll, lifting the head and tail. [*4 times*]

Tip: *This fluid movement begins at the end of the tailbone and rolls through your spine, like a wave that crests behind the heart.*

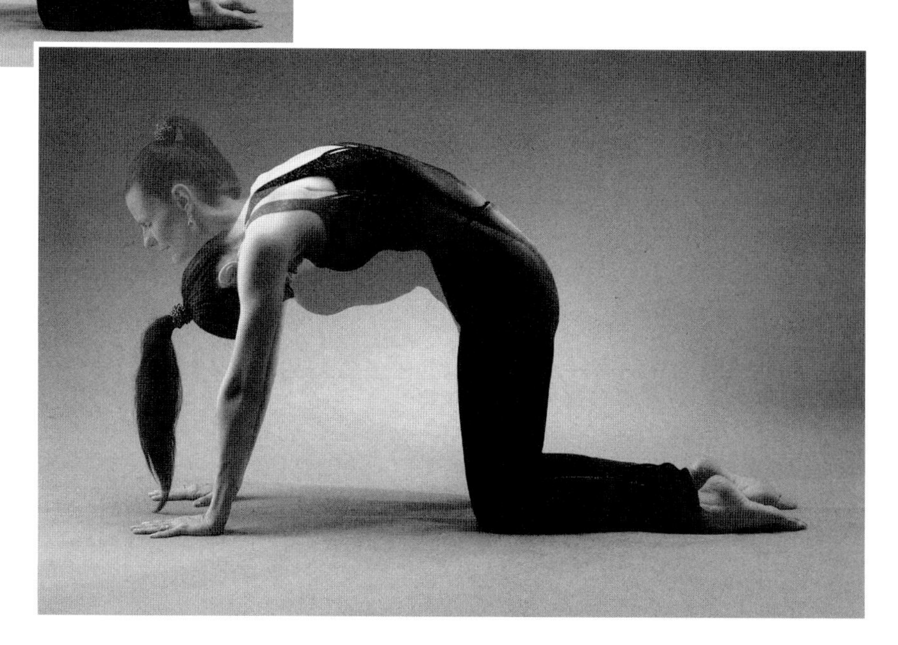

GENTLE VERSIONS

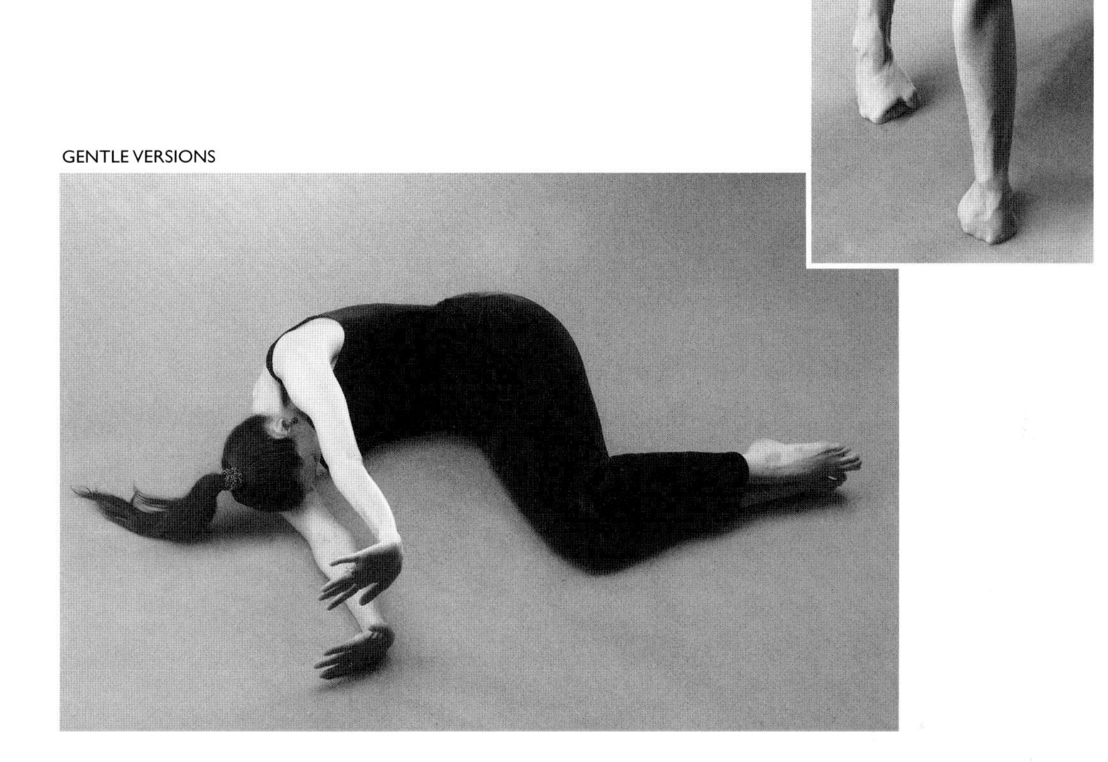

Gentle Versions: *If this position hurts your wrists, rise up on your fists. If your knees are an issue, turn on your side and mimic the pose by bending the knees hip-high and extending the arms in front of your shoulders. Inhale to prepare, then exhale and do the same spine-rolling motion, from the tail upward through lower, middle, and upper back.*

16. Table Pushups

[for biceps, triceps, pectorals]

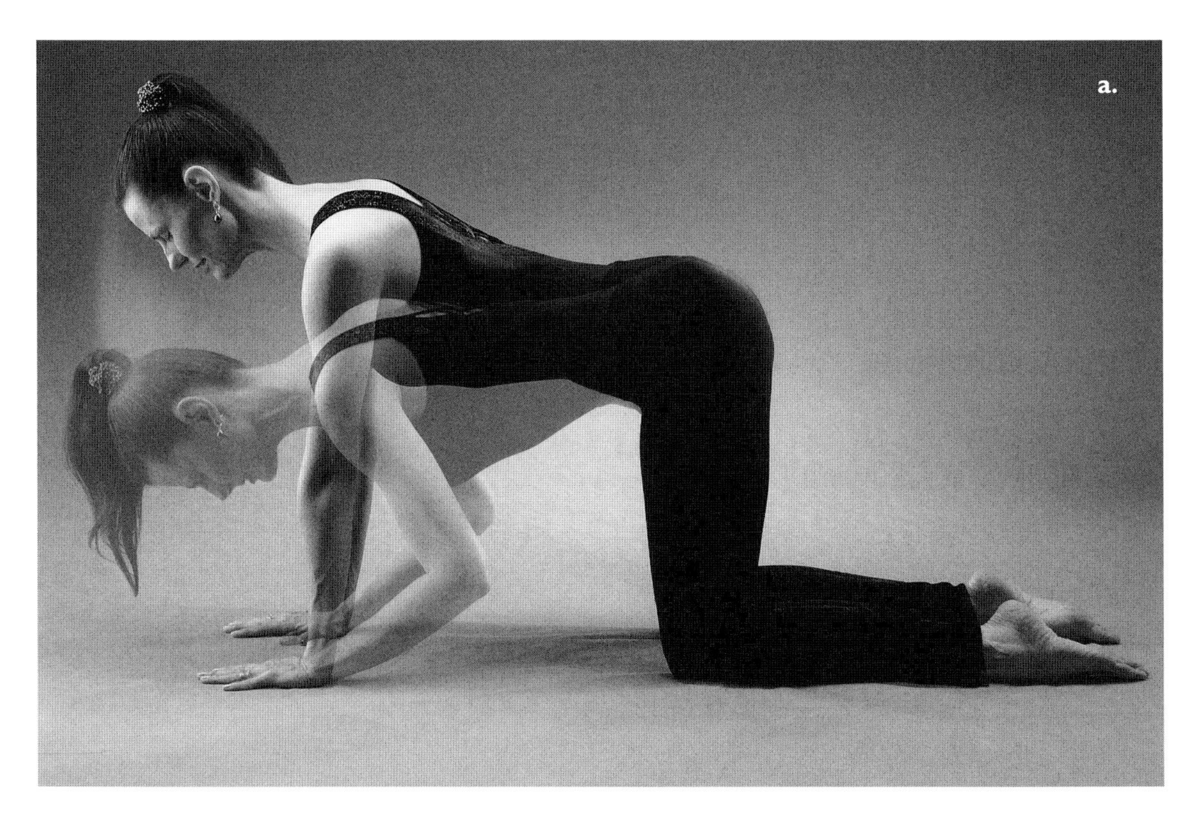

PREPARATION

Remaining on your hands and knees, flatten your back so that you could serve a meal on it.

MOTION

a. Inhale and bend the arms, lowering the upper body toward the floor. Exhale and straighten the arms, remembering to travel the path as you breathe. [*4 times, then, staying down with arms bent, 16 pulses, exhaling with each pulse.*]

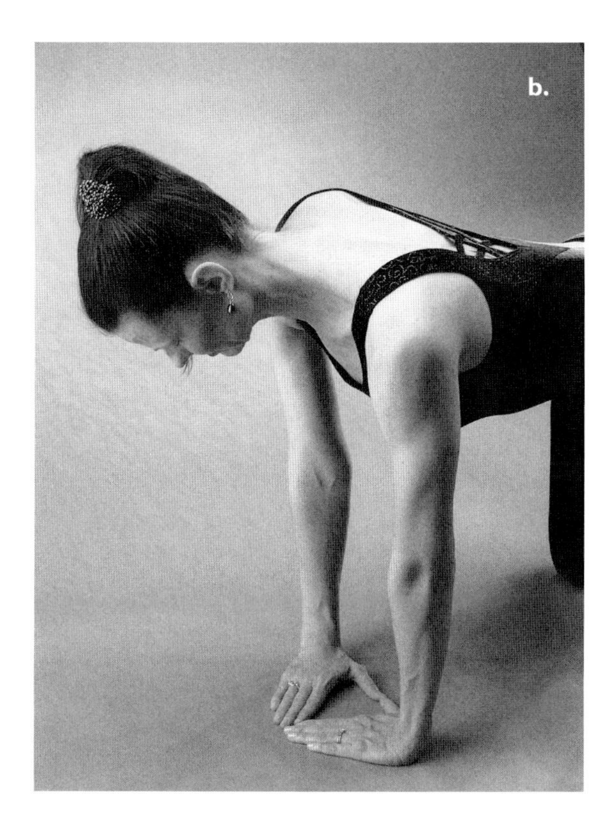

b. Repeat the sequence, but with your hands together, the tips of your thumbs and forefingers meeting in a triangle under the heart center. [*4 times, followed by 16 pulses*]

Tip: *Keep your back straight, head in line with spine (not dropped toward the floor).*

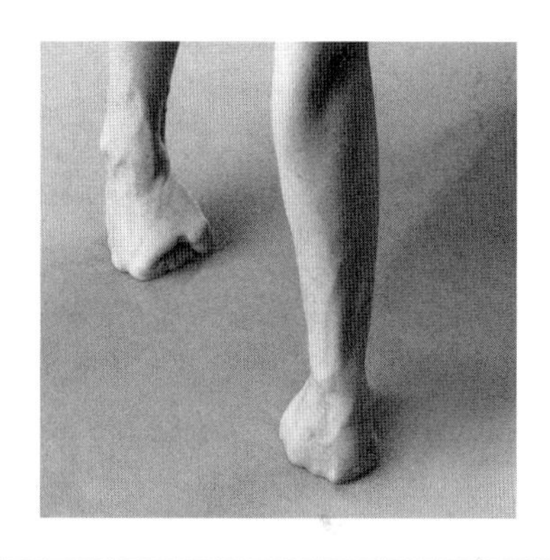

Gentle Version: *If this hurts your wrists, get up on your fists.*

17. Baby Pose

[for spine, digestion, low-back pain]

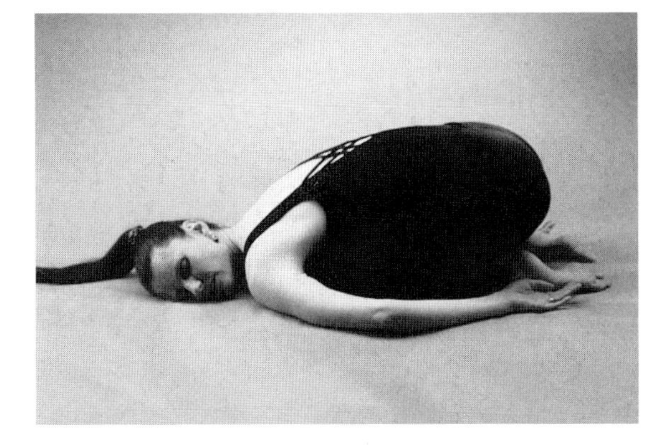

PREPARATION

Sit back on your heels, legs hip-width apart so that the belly and chest can fall between your thighs. Rest your head comfortably (on either the brow or cheek) and place your arms at your sides, the shoulders waterfalling off your spine. Make yourself at home, as wise babies do.

Breathing Pattern

Whatever position you've chosen, get comfortable. We'll spend about a minute here, aiming the breath into different parts of the back.

a. Inhale and visualize yourself breathing directly into your *upper back,* filling the shoulders and shoulder blades with wind. Exhale and relax.

b. Now move into the *middle back,* inhaling and feeling it swell in response. Exhale, drifting down.

c. Traveling to the *lower back* now, inhale and fill the lumbar chamber with light and wind. Exhale and relax.

d. Lower now, breathe directly into your *hips and pelvis.* Exhale and rest.

e. Now, breathing into the *whole surface of the back,* inhale and feel it rise like a great silken parachute, billowing in the wind. Exhale, feeling it drift back to earth. [*2 breaths*]

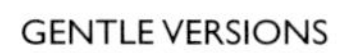
GENTLE VERSIONS

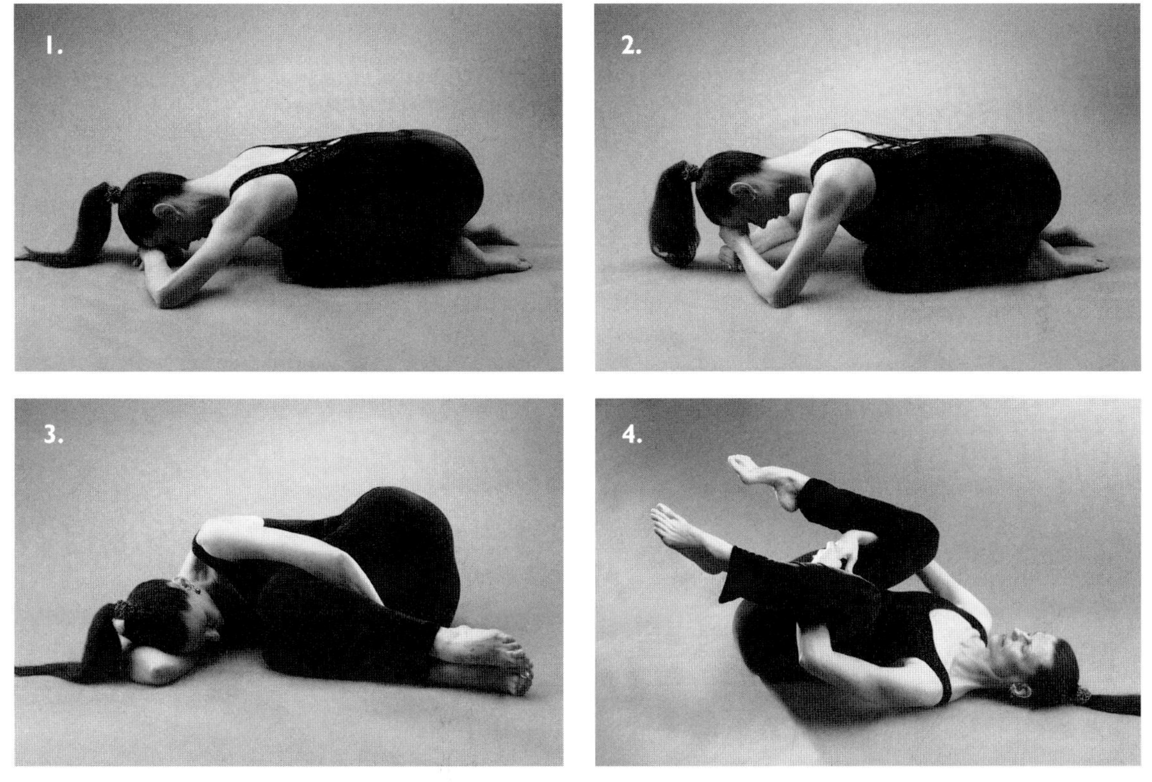

Gentle Versions: *If your hips are more than three inches from your heels, place your hands (or fists) under the brow and ease the hips down toward your heels (figures 1 and 2). If your knees are an issue, turn on your side in fetal position and do the breathing from here (figure 3). If you prefer, turn over on your back and rest in Double Leg Press (figure 4).*

18. Railroad

[full body stretch]

PREPARATION

Gently rolling over on your back, stretch the arms overhead and the legs out below, as if you were an endless pair of railroad tracks. Let the palms look up at the sky and the soles down at the earth. Inhale, re-establishing the path.

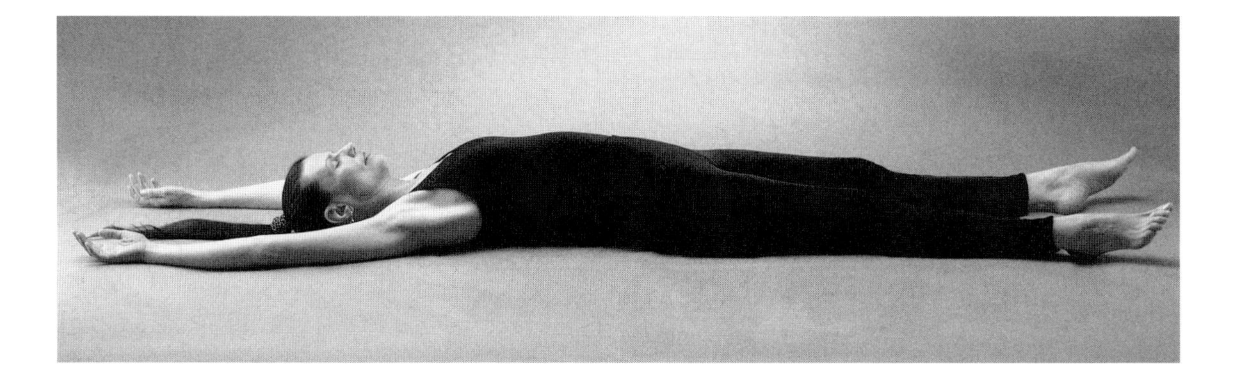

MOTION

Exhale, pushing your fingers and toes out of the belly, toward opposite horizons, elongating everything. [*3 breaths*]

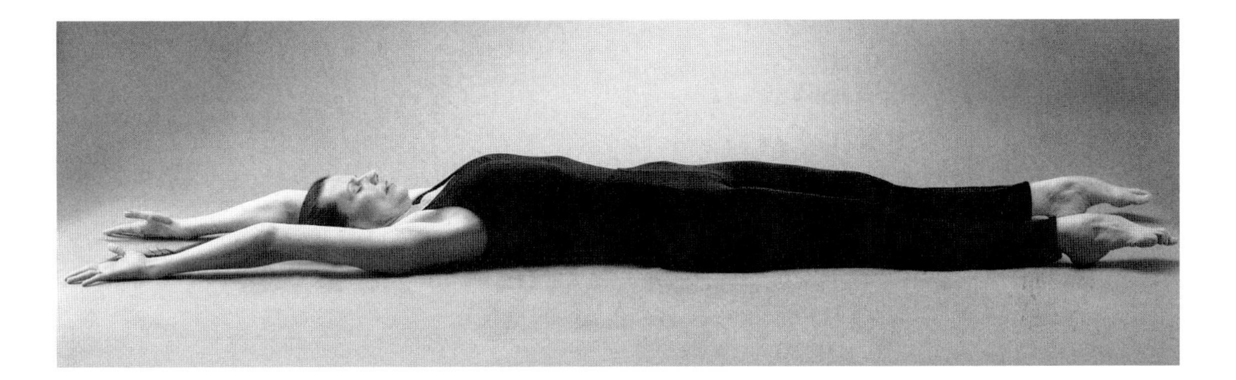

19. Tail Curls/Wing Lifts

[for abdominals]

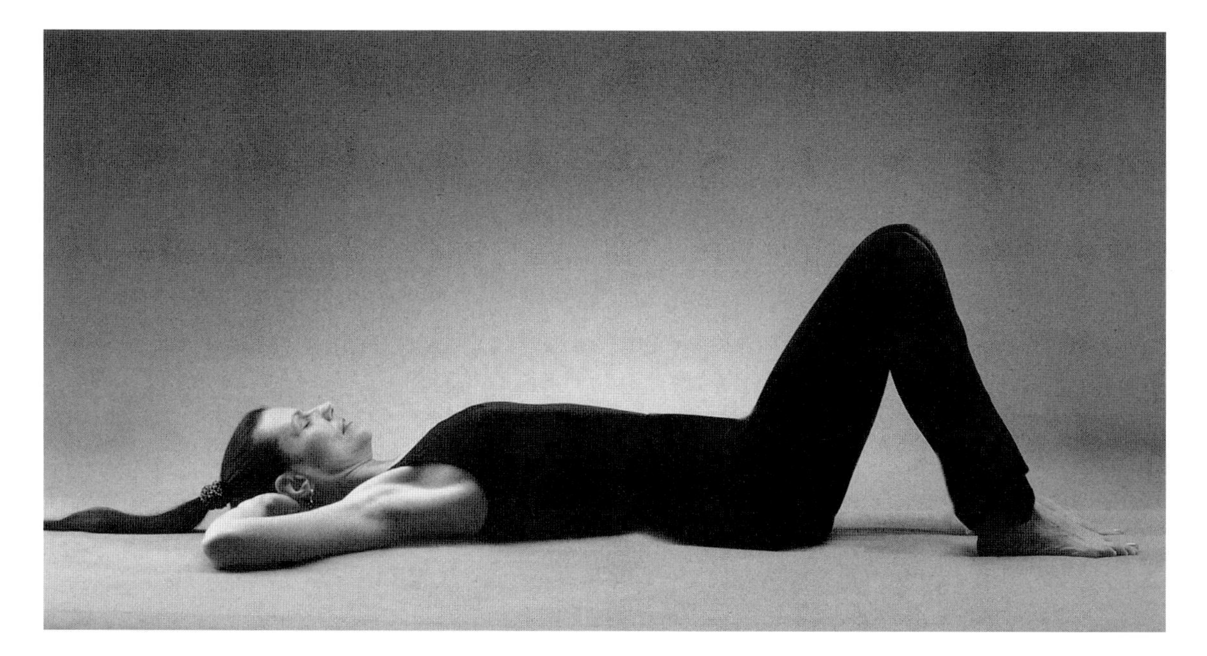

PREPARATION

Bending your knees, plant your feet hip-width apart on the floor and lace the fingers behind your head. Inhale, filling the belly.

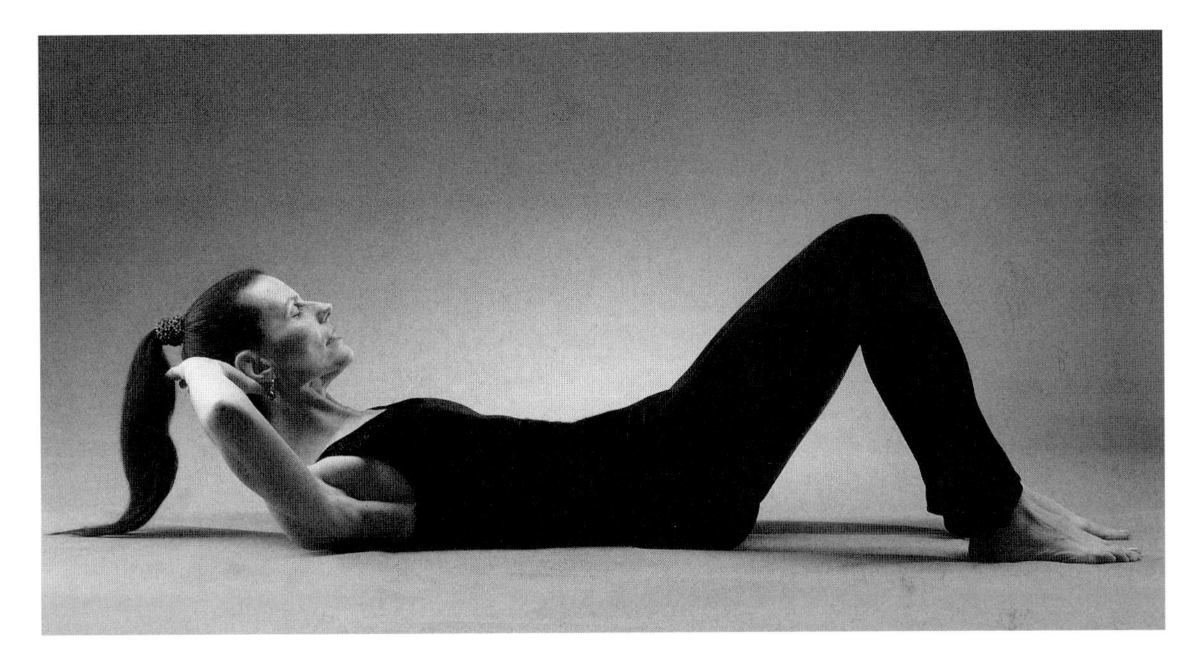

MOTION

Exhale as you (1) curl the tail, (2) empty the belly, and (3) lift the wings (shoulder blades) off the floor, feeling the flow of the exhalation through the heart. Inhale and unroll. [*4 times slow, then 16–32 pulses*]

Tip: *Keep the elbows wide, and source the head in the belly, not the neck. Aim to get your wings off the floor by lifting from behind the heart. As the upper body lifts, do not "grip" the belly; it must soften and fall as the head rises.*

20. Corpse Pose

[for relaxation, realignment, rejuvenation]

To finish, we return to where we started. Let your legs stream out, hip-width apart, arms 45 degrees from the sides of your body. Notice how different the body feels from when you first took this position—how much more of you is present, and how much more space there is to be present in. Inhale downward, feeling how the path has cleared and lengthened.

Exhale and return along the spine through the heart, the abdominals sweetly married to the wind. Continue path breathing for as long as you like, assimilating all that the body has undergone. After a while, let go of the breath and just feel the body, basking in your own radiance, like the light that moves beyond the lampshade and into the world.

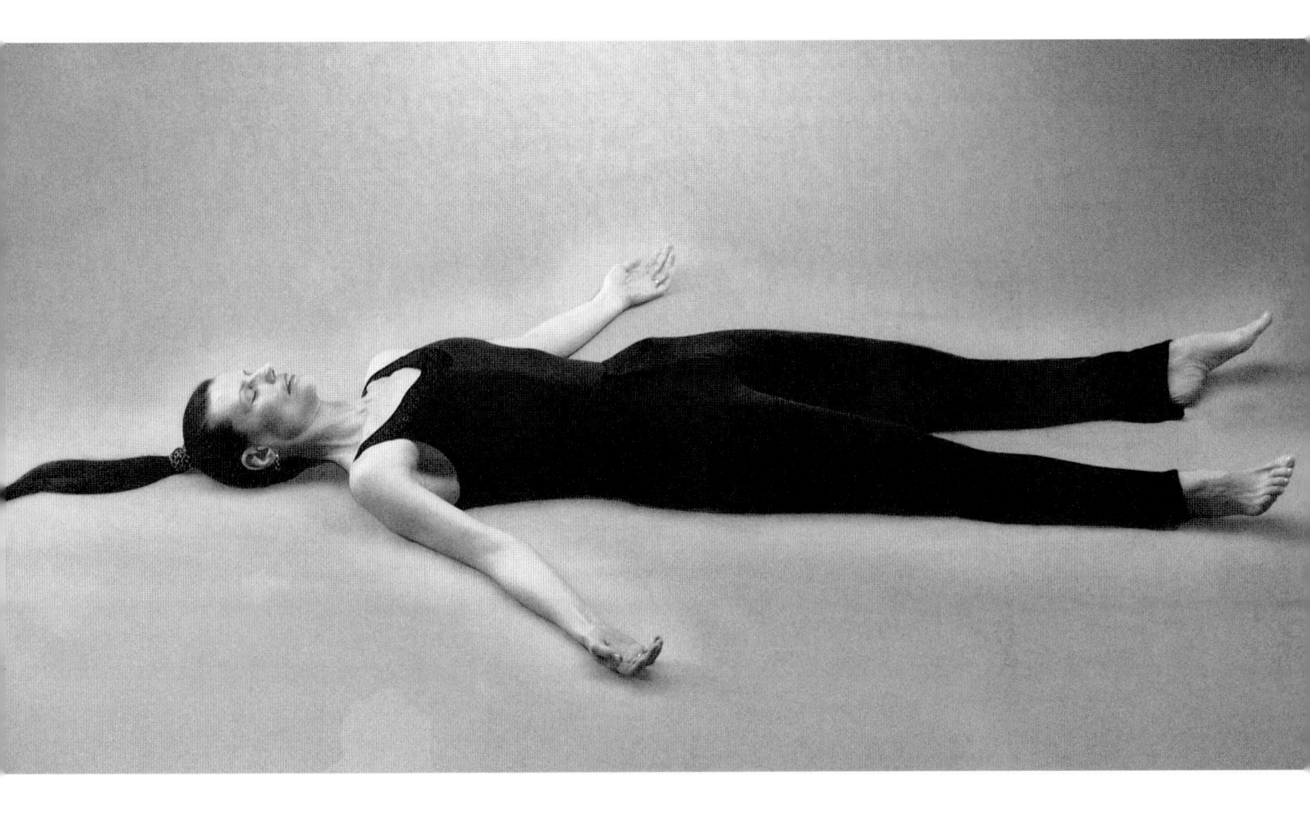

Yoganetics for Beginners: Flow Chart

Condensed Photo-Map of the Workout

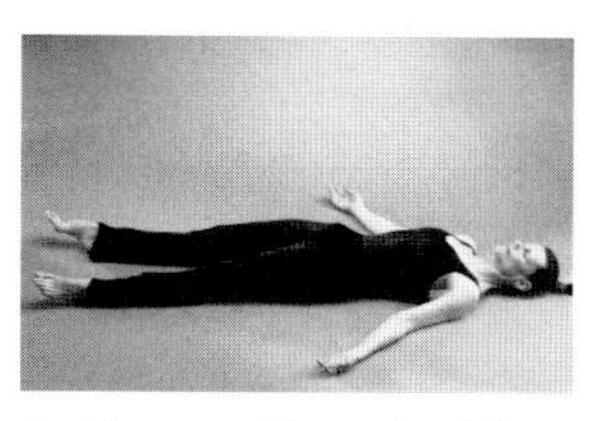

1. Corpse Pose (p. 46) [*5-minute voyage, 8 path breaths*]

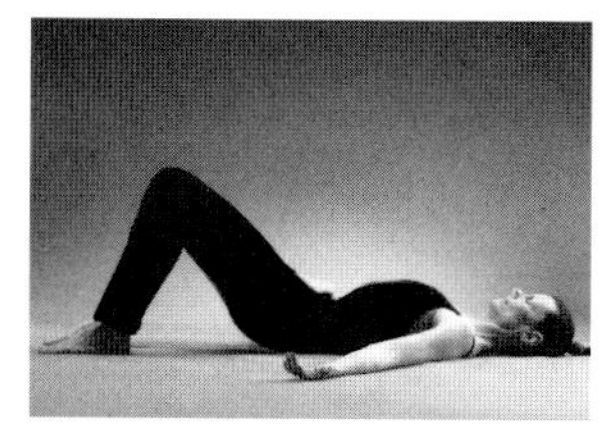

2. Tail Curls (p. 48) [*8 times*]

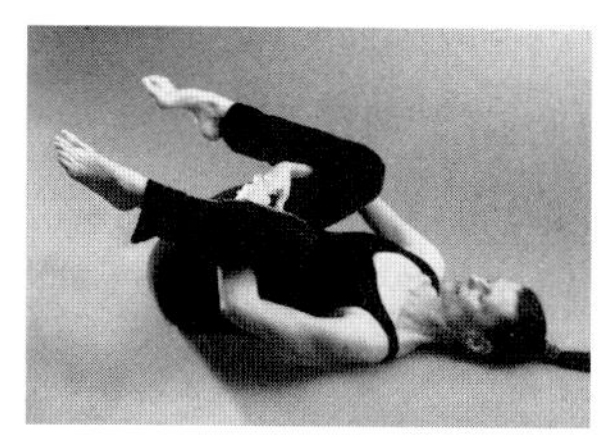

3. Double Leg Press (p. 50) [*4 breaths*]

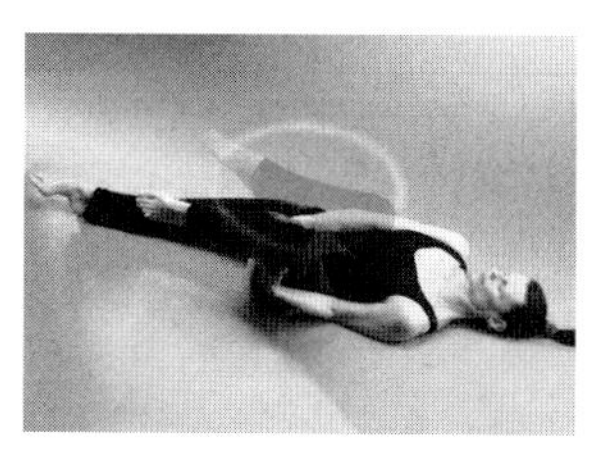

4. Thigh Circles (p. 52) [*4 times, then reverse*]

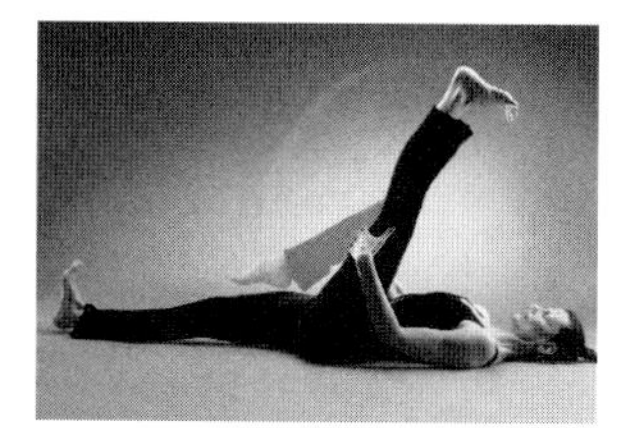

5. Separated Leg Push (p. 54) [*4 times*]

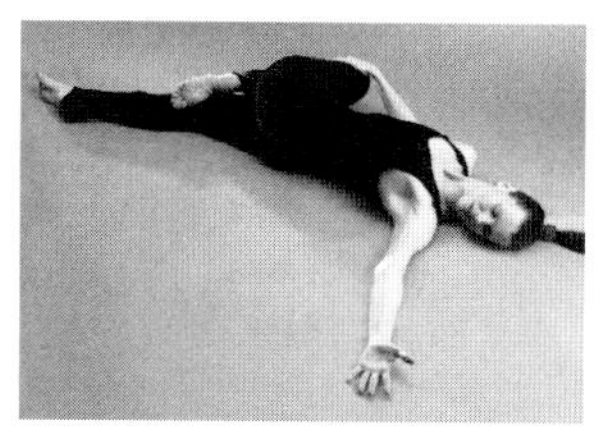

6. Supported Single Legovers (p. 56) [*3 breaths*]

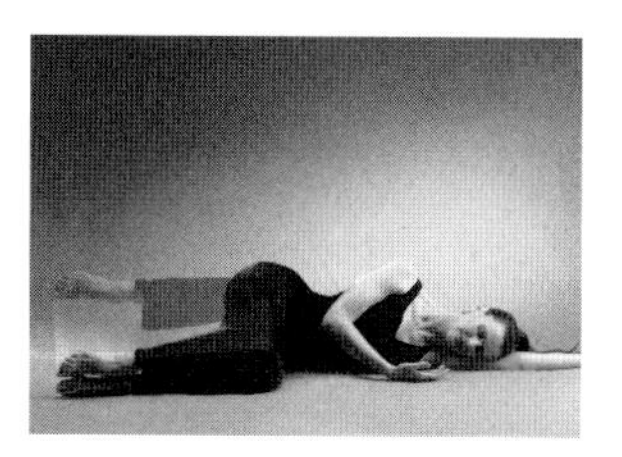

7. Groaner (p. 58) [*(a) 4 to 8 times, 16 pulses; (b) 4 to 8 times, 16 pulses*]

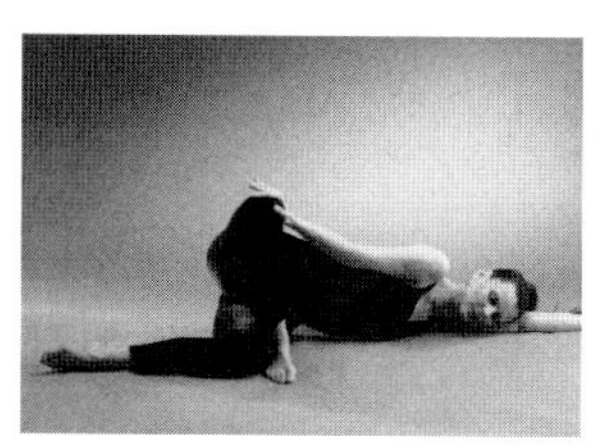

8. Barn Door (p. 60) [*3 breaths*]

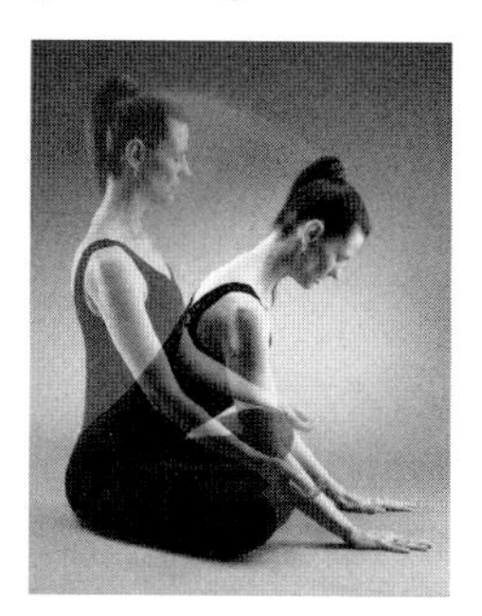

9. Easy Flatback (p. 62) [*4 breaths center, 2 breaths left, 2 breaths right*]

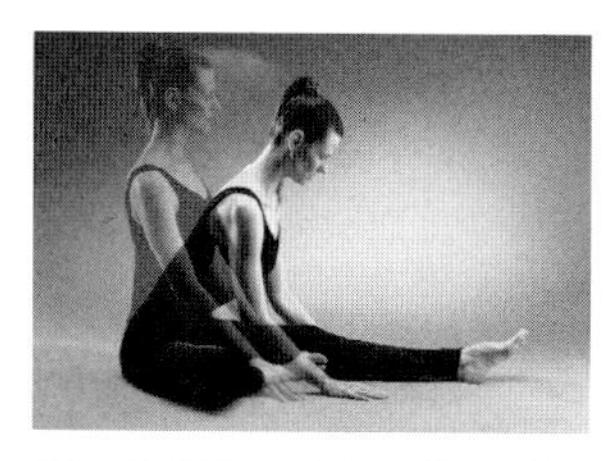

10. Folding Tree (p. 64) [*3 breaths*]

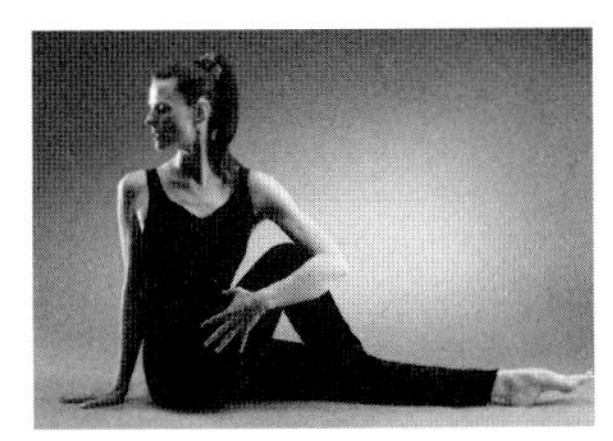

11. Tree Spiral (p. 66)
[*3 breaths*]

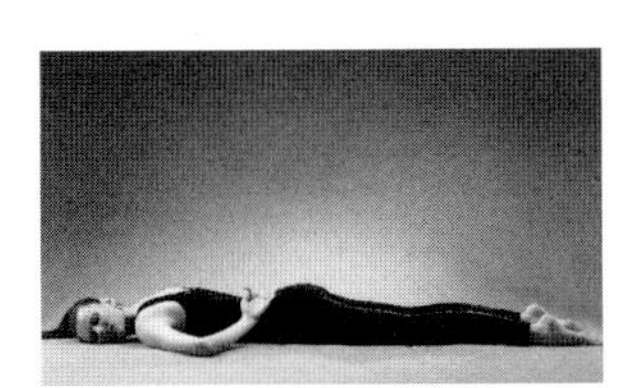

12. Rear Window (p. 68)
[*4 breaths*]

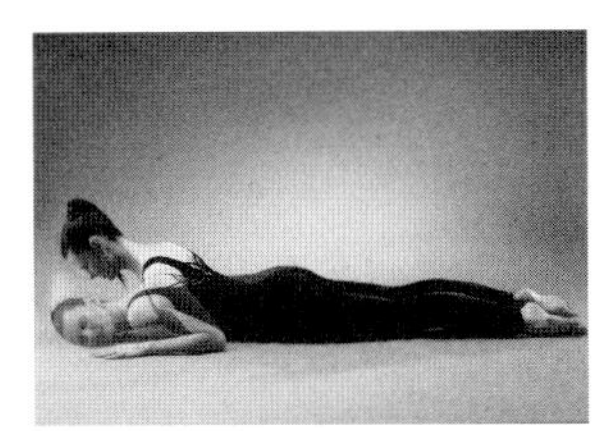

13. Pre-Cobra (p. 70)
[*4 times*]

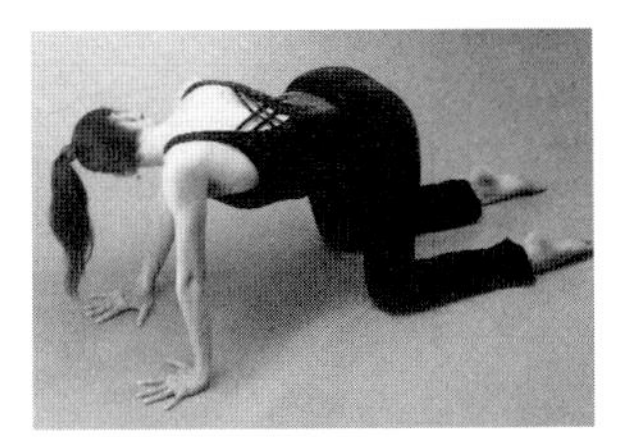

14. Lateral Cat (p. 72)
[*4 times, alternating left and right*]

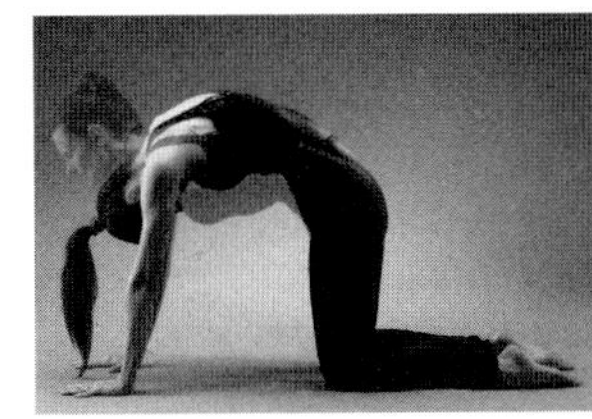

15. Cat (p. 74)
[*4 times*]

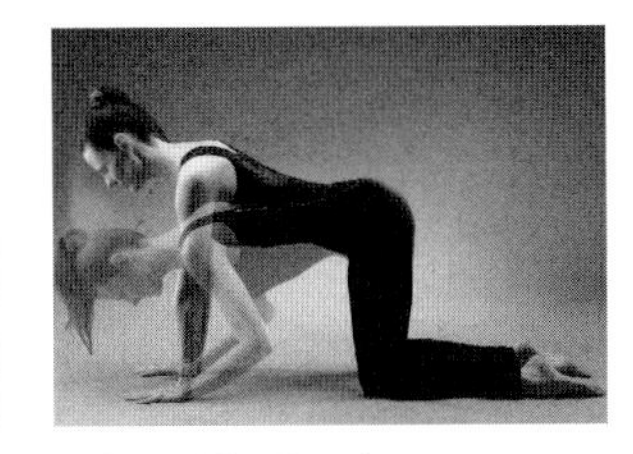

16. Table Pushups (p. 76) [*(a) 4 times, 16 pulses; (b) 4 times, 16 pulses*]

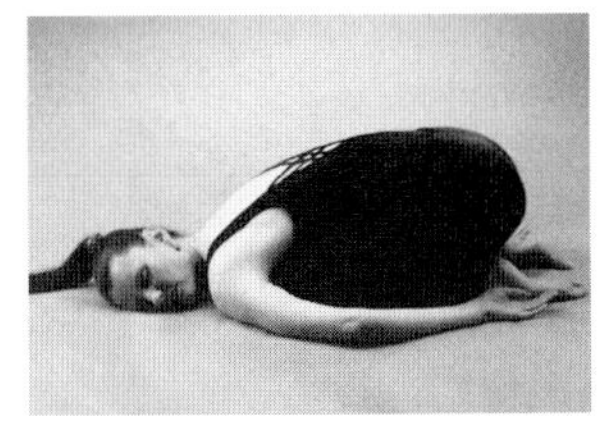

17. Baby Pose (p. 78)
[*4 exploring breaths; 2 whole-back breaths*]

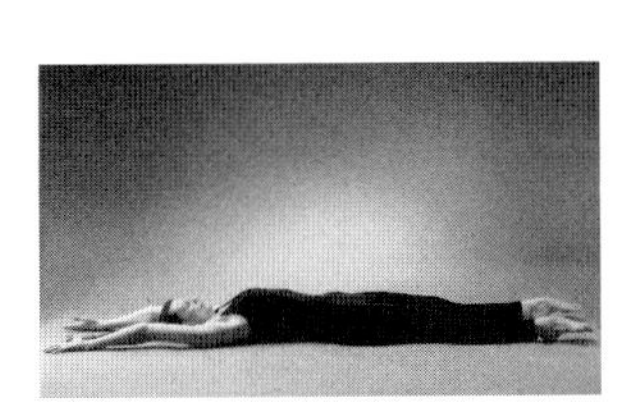

18. Railroad (p. 80)
[*3 breaths*]

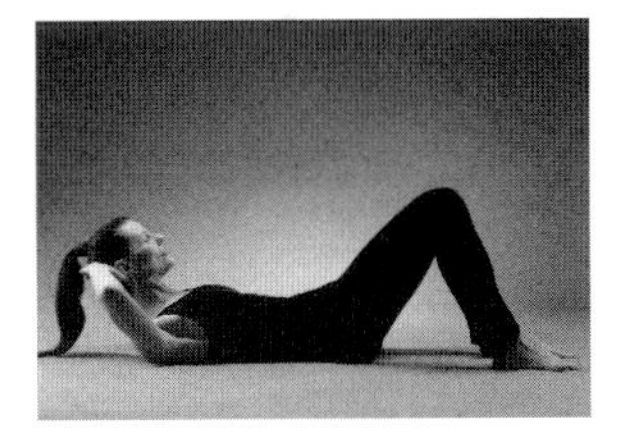

19. Tail Curls/Wing Lifts (p. 82) [*4 times, 16–32 pulses*]

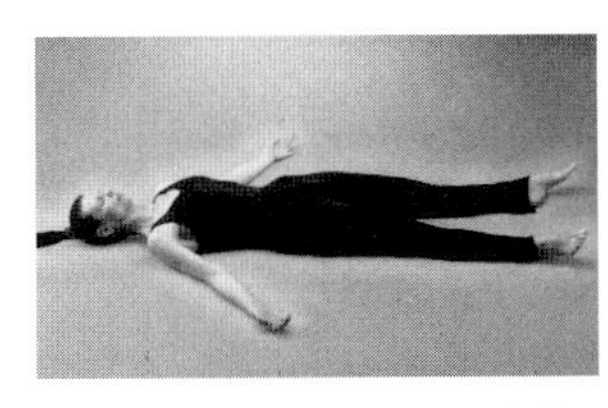

20. Corpse Pose (p. 84)
[*meditation*]

Seven

Yoganetics for Intermediate Students

"I must follow my thread," returned Irene, "whatever I do."

GEORGE MACDONALD, *THE PRINCESS AND THE GOBLIN*

When should you move from the beginner to the intermediate workout? That's of course up to you, your body, and the state of your practice. Generally, beginners are beginners for more than a few weeks or months. If, after six months of twice-weekly training, you feel ready—or if you are already advanced in another technique and have moved through the beginner workout for a while—you may want to begin the intermediate level, modifying as needed along the way. (Advanced workouts will appear in the next book, *Advanced Yoganetics*.)

I am an eternal beginner. After decades of immersion in this work, I still return to beginner workouts as the foundation on which all higher floors depend with their far-flung balconies and views. If the groundwork is not done, the house, however fancy, will not stand. If you have built a strong foundation, then you can set foot on the curving staircases.

Always review the Ground Rules (pp. 43–44) before you practice.

---

1. Corpse Pose

[for relaxation, realignment, rejuvenation]

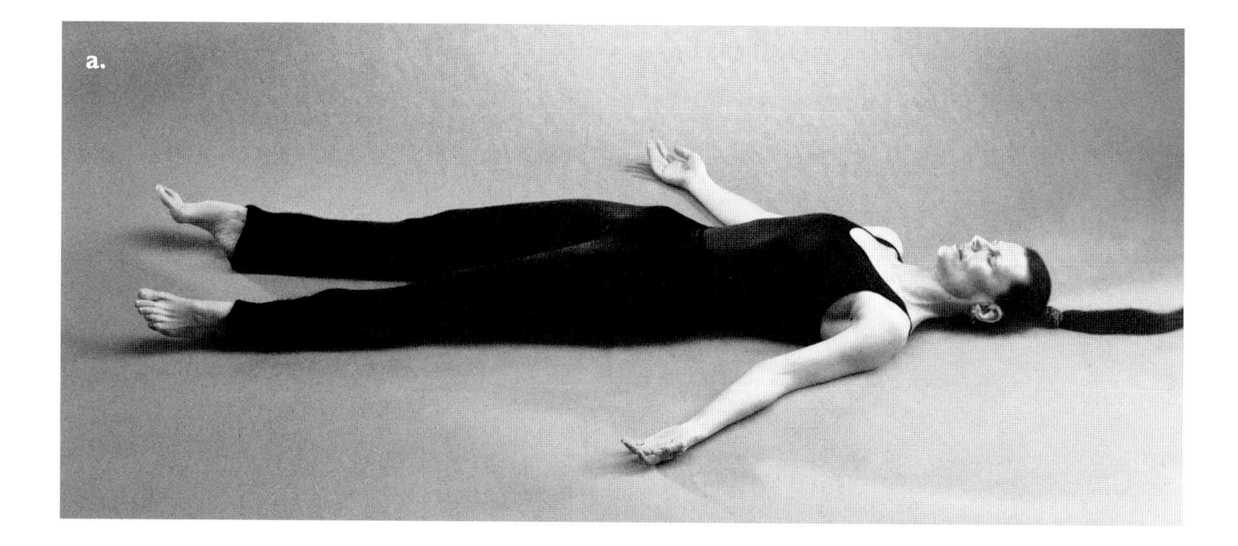

a. *The Voyage:* Sprawl on your back, legs hip-width apart, arms 45 degrees from your sides, palms up. Relax the shoulders and lengthen the secondary curves of the spine—behind the neck and waist. Sink into the earth that cradles you. Close your eyes and take the voyage, gliding through the body from the crown of your head through the soles of your feet, lingering anywhere you feel discomfort or a blockage of flow. [*5 minutes*]

Gentle Version: *Bend your knees and plant your feet on the floor hip-width apart.*

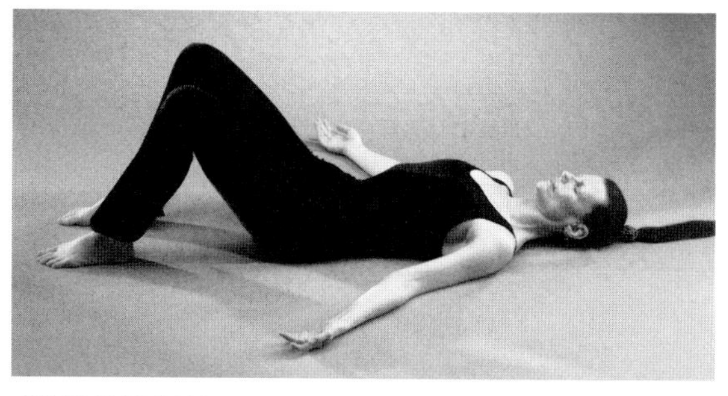

GENTLE VERSION

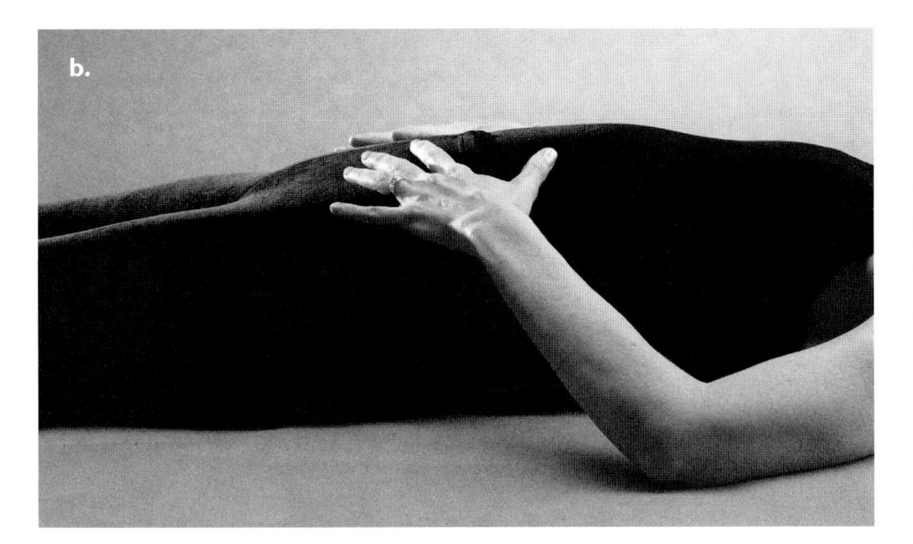

Inhale
Follow the wind down the path to explore the cave.

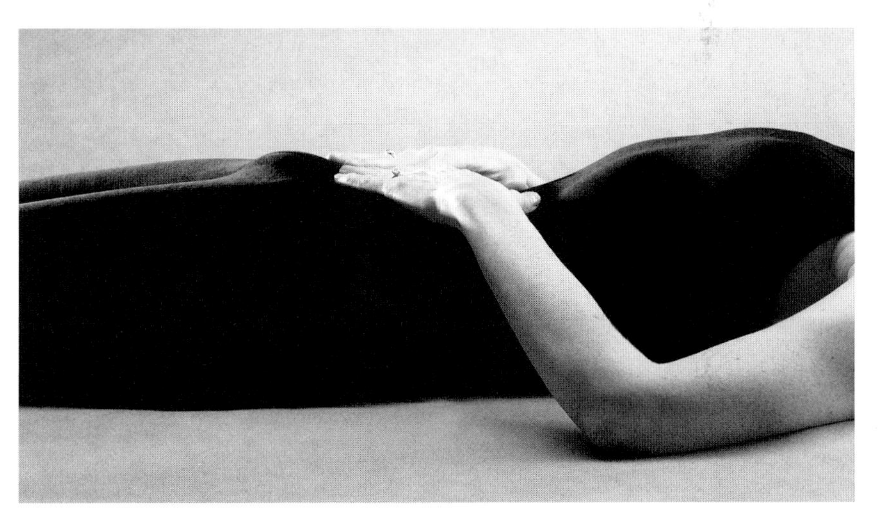

Exhale
Follow the wind along the path back through the heart.

b. *The Path [for lungs, abdominals, reintegration]*: Return your attention to the heart. Travel the path of breath along the spine between the heart center and the gravitational center, moving downward as you inhale to fill the belly, and upward as you exhale, the belly falling as it follows through. [*8 slow breaths*]

2. Tail Curls

[for abdominals, inner thighs, hamstrings, spine]

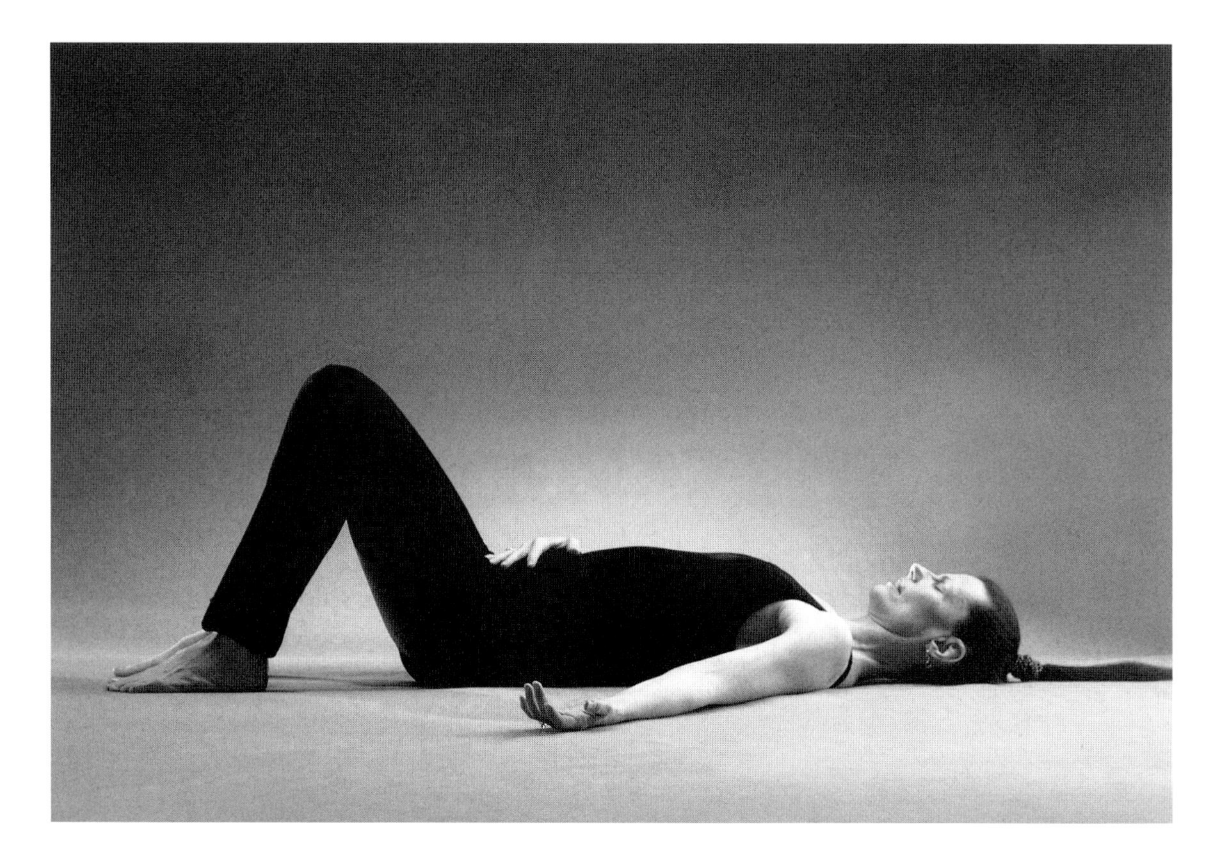

PREPARATION

Bend your knees and plant your feet on the floor hip-width apart, parallel with each other. Inhale, feeling the wind move down the path to the backmost corners of the cave.

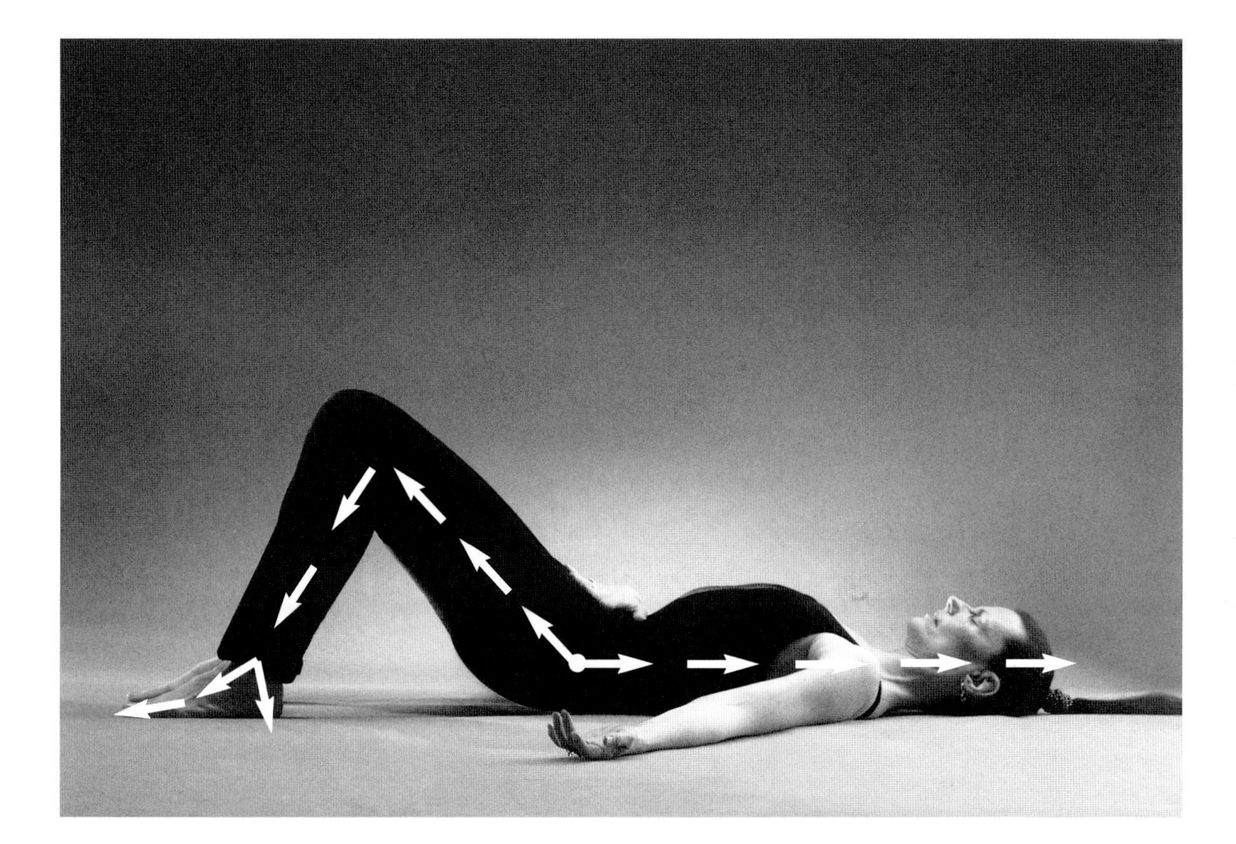

MOTION

Exhale, rooting through all ten toes as you curl your tailbone slightly up toward the sky. Feel how the belly is drawn along the spine on the exhalation. Inhale, filling the cave as the tail unrolls to earth. [*8 times*]

Tip: *During each Tail Curl, feel the rich opposition of the feet pushing down and the crown of the head pushing up, out of the core.*

3. Double Legovers

[for abdominals, spine]

PREPARATION

Walk the feet and legs together. Gently let the knees fall to one side, the head looking the other way. Feet stay in touch with the floor, knees glued together. Inhale, expanding the belly.

Tip: *Take the knees only as far to the side as they can go without separating.*

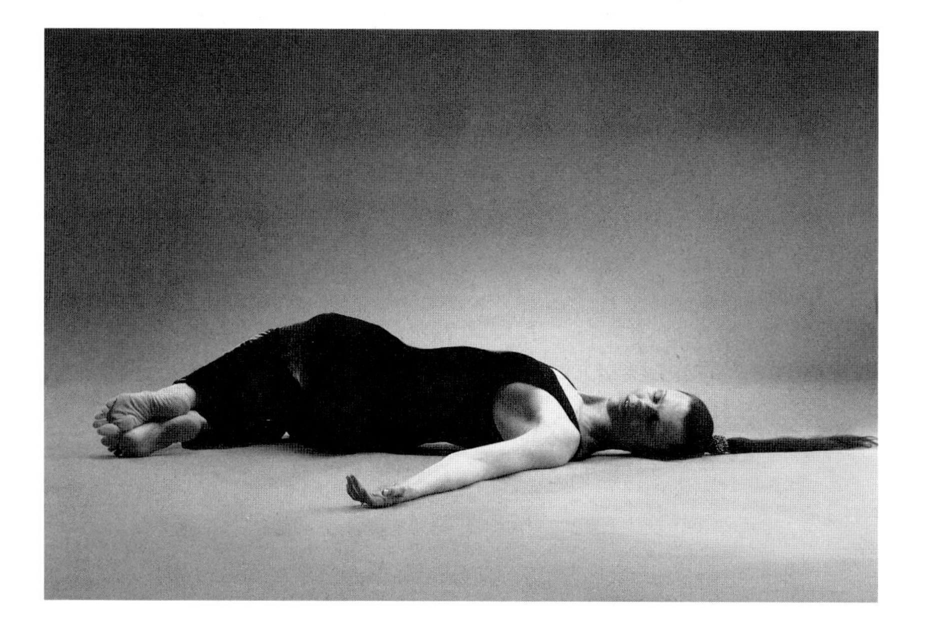

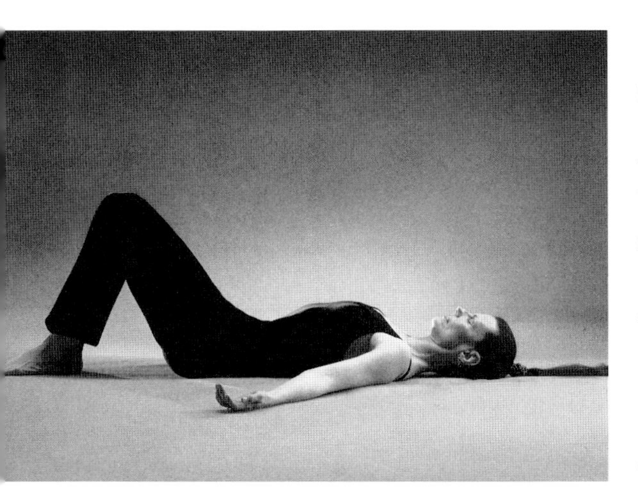

MOTION

Exhale, using the breath and belly to pull the thighs back to center as slowly as you dare. Roll back and forth over the hips this way in ultra-slow motion. [*6 times, alternating left and right*]

***Tip:** Don't push with the bottom thigh to center the legs. The work is wholly abdominal, and tied to the exhalation.*

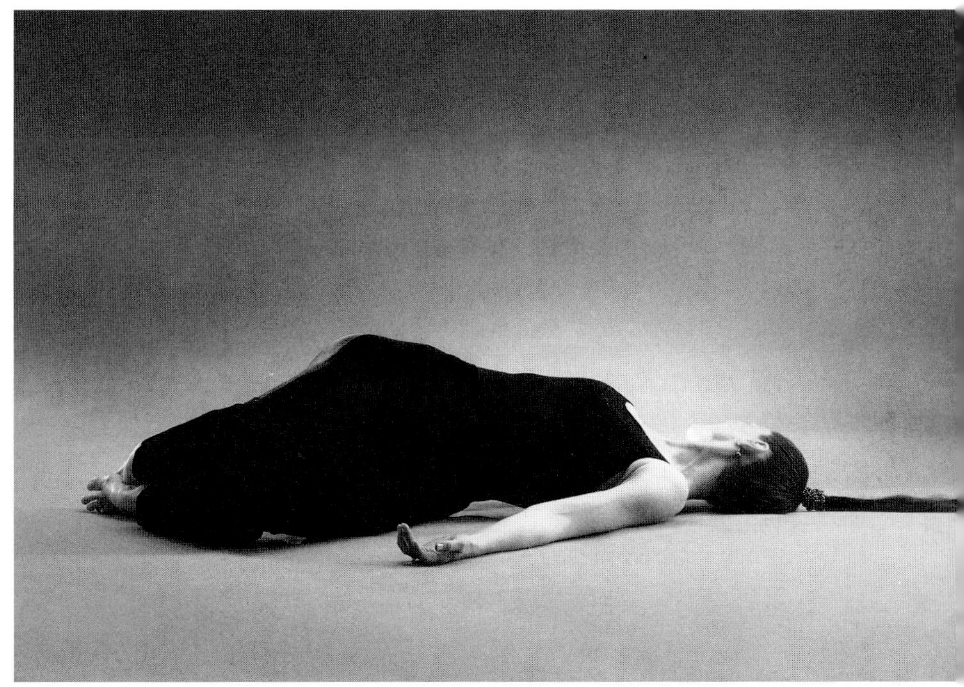

4. Double Leg Press

[for spine, digestion, circulation]

PREPARATION

Bring the knees to the chest and hold hands behind the backs of your thighs, legs hip-width apart. Drop your chin and lengthen the back of the neck. Keep the hips on the floor and feel the lower back spreading open. Inhale, breathing downward into the belly, pelvis, and seat.

Gentle Version: *Hold the backs of your thighs separately, hip-width apart.*

MOTION

Exhale, following the underground river of wind along the spine. As the belly gets out of the way, your legs will fall naturally closer to the body. [*4 breaths*]

Tip: *Relax your shoulders throughout.*

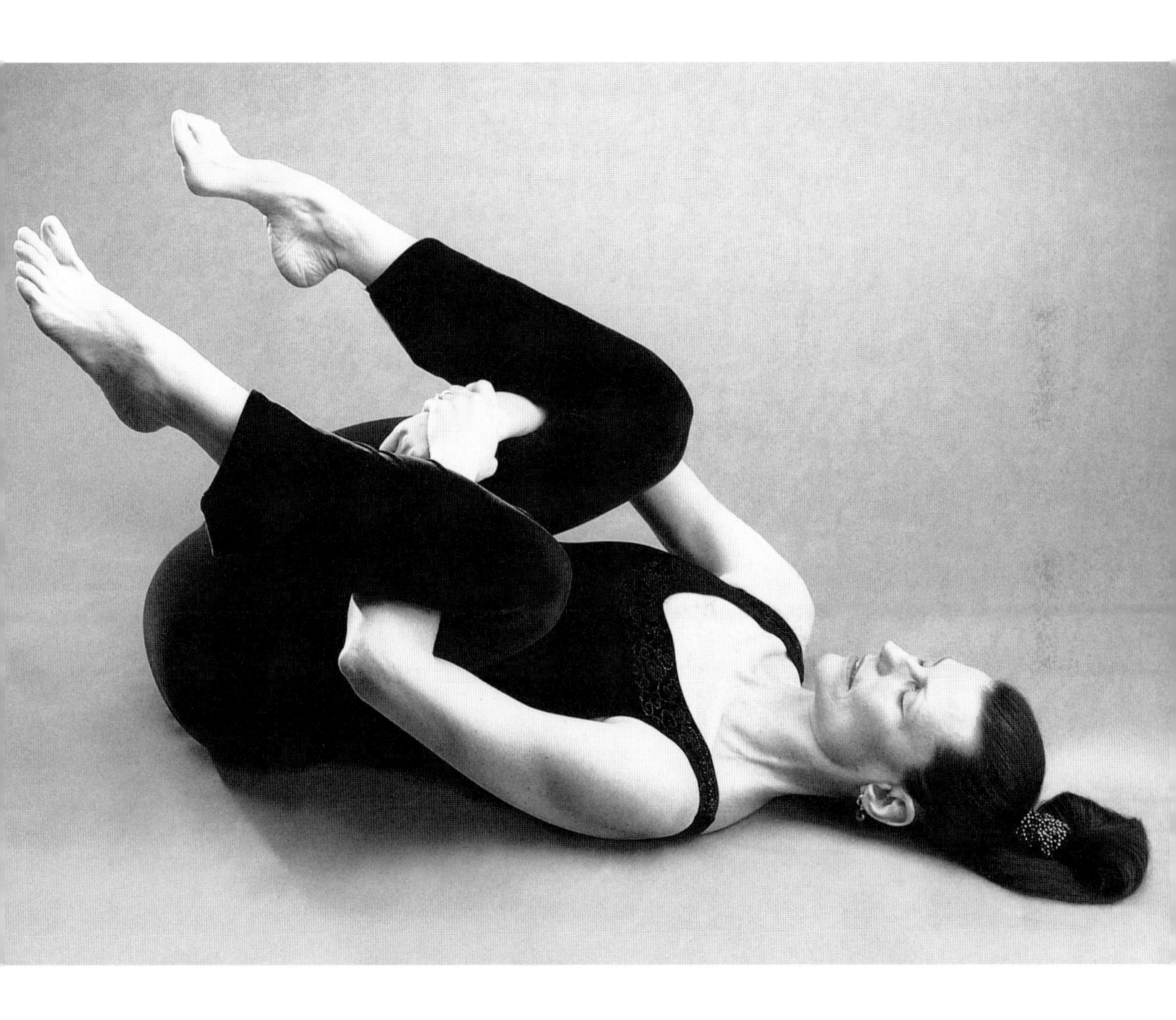

5. Double Leg Push

[for arms, spine, belly, legs]

PREPARATION

Separate the hands to hold the backs of your thighs, legs hip-width apart. Inhale, filling the belly.

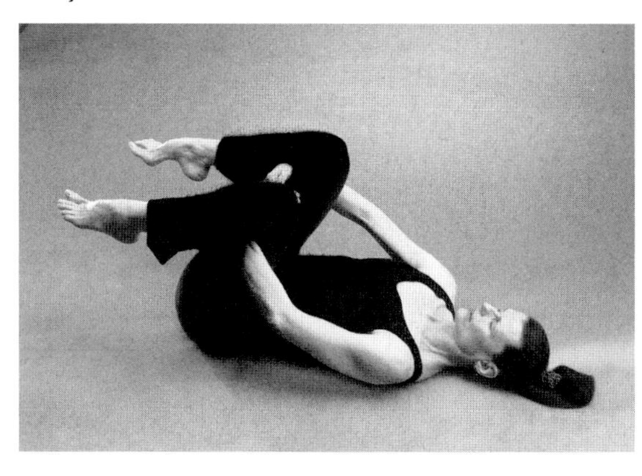

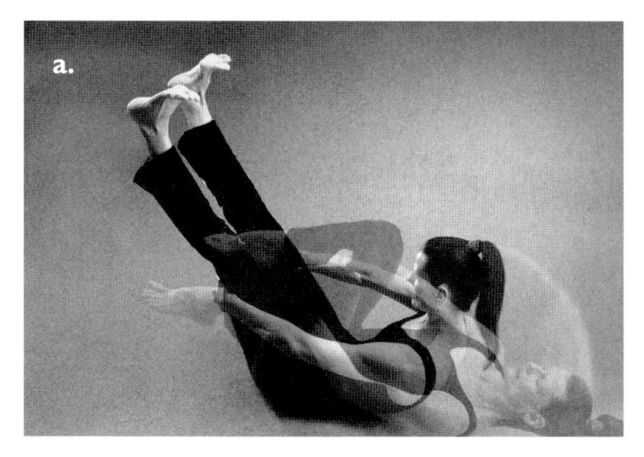

MOTION

a. Exhale and push the head and heels out of the belly, straightening your legs below hip level and rounding the arms to lift the upper body off the floor. Inhale and return, unrolling the back of the neck to the earth by drawing in the chin and pointing through the eartips. [*2 times*]

Tip: *The lower back stays on the floor throughout. Let the arms do the work here, so that the belly can easily fall on exhalation as the head rises.*

---

c. Exhale and repeat, this time turning the legs out, like a dancer, and pressing the inner thighs together. [2 *times*]

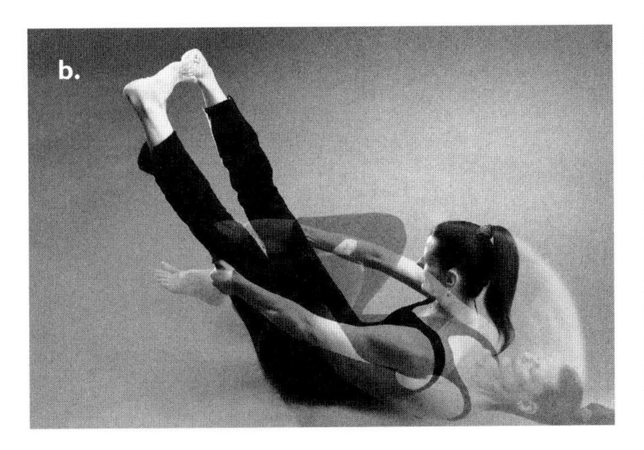

b. Exhale and repeat, this time turning the legs inward, pigeon-toed. [2 *times*]

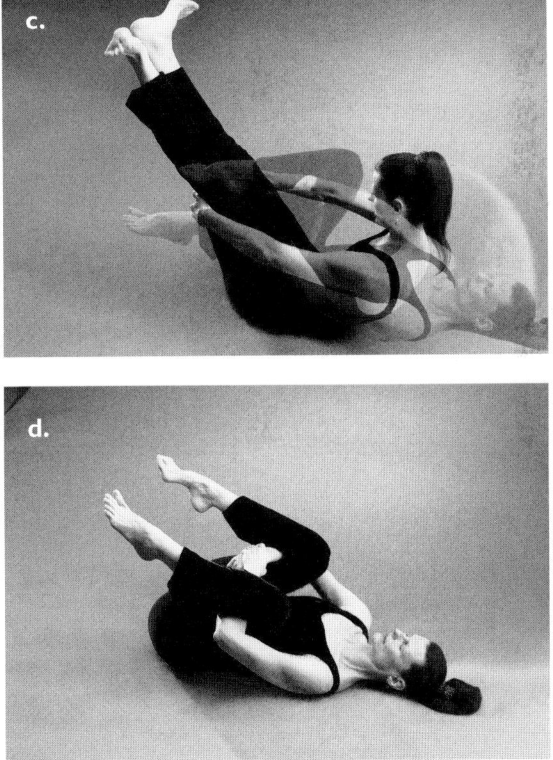

d. Inhale and return, finishing in Double Leg Press. Rest.

6. Separated Leg Push, with Dive

[for hamstrings, quadriceps, calves, inner thighs, spine]

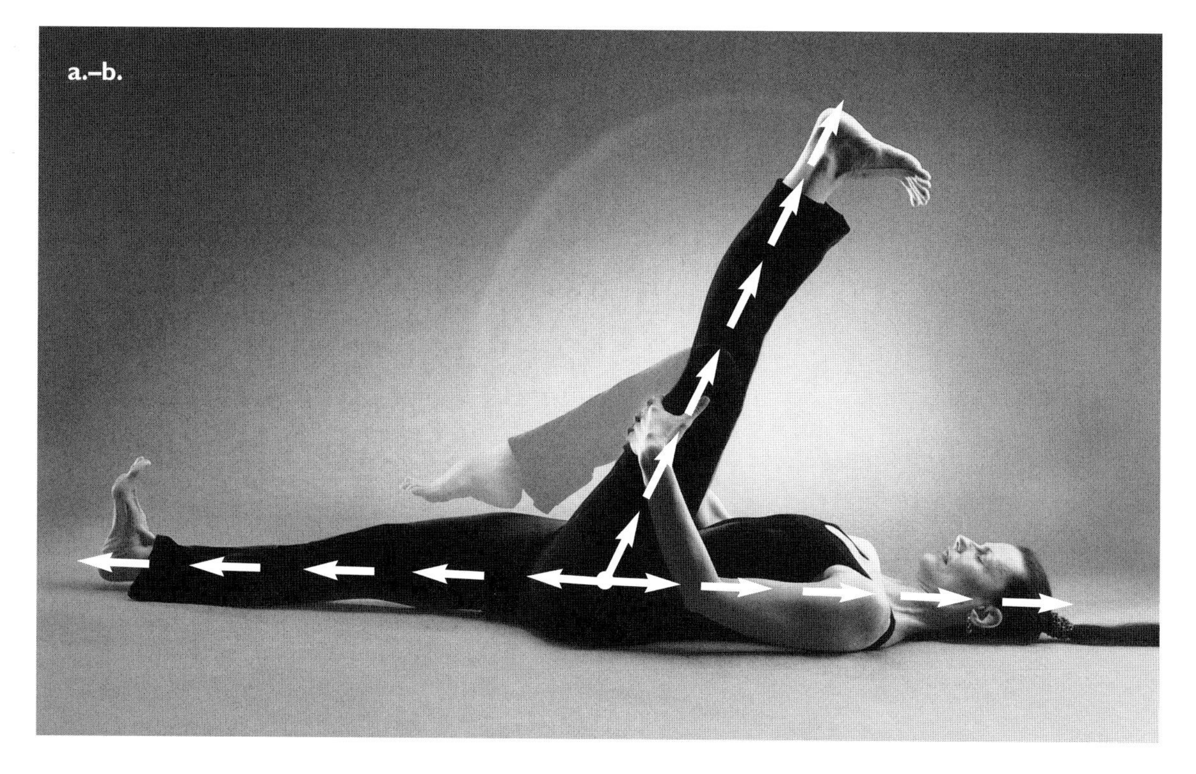

PREPARATION

Bend your knee (left first) and hold the thigh, the other leg extended on the floor. Inhale, expanding the belly.

MOTION

a. Exhale, flexing the feet and extending both legs straight, pushing the top heel into the sky, sending heels and head equally and endlessly out of the cave. Feel the belly fall as the wind flows up the spine. Inhale and return, bending the top knee. [*2 times*]

b. Exhale, flexing the feet and extending both legs. This time linger here, with straight legs, to follow the path of breath along the spine. [*2 breaths*]

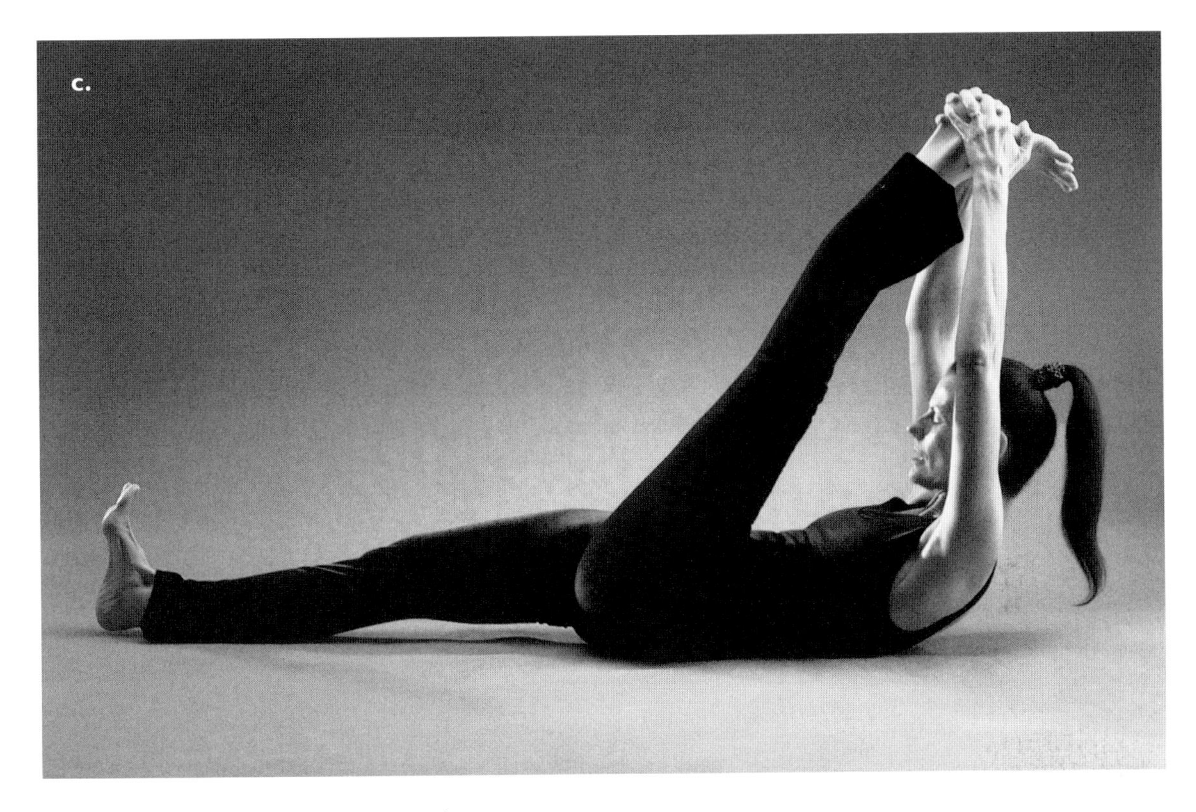

c. If your top leg is not yet straight, remain with your head and shoulders on the floor and simply breathe. If the leg you're holding is straight, exhale and extend through your crown, lifting the upper body off the floor. Climb your hands up your extended leg to a comfortable position, keeping the shoulders down. Rest here and breathe, filling the cave and traveling the path. [*2 long breaths*] Inhale and return, drawing in the chin, rolling through the back of your neck to earth. [*Do exercises 7 and 8 before switching sides.*]

Gentle Version: *Bend the standing leg and plant the foot on the floor, keeping this leg bent throughout.*

GENTLE VERSION

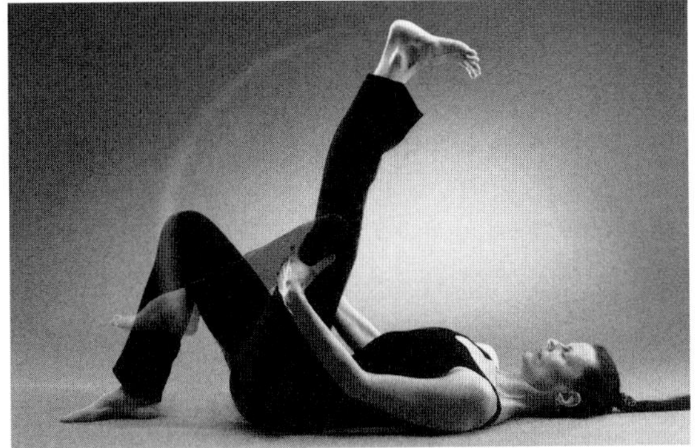

7. Yoga Zip-ups

[for upper and lower abdominals, thighs]

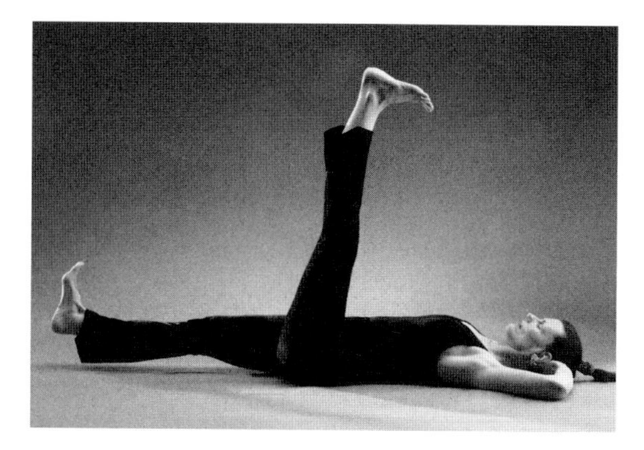

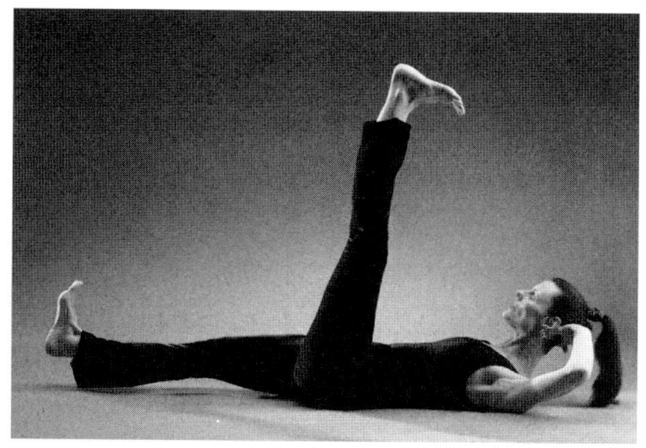

PREPARATION

Still with the leg extended above your body, interlace the fingers behind the head, and raise your standing leg three inches from the floor. Inhale, allowing the belly to expand.

MOTION

Exhale and slowly lift your wings (shoulder blades) off the floor, the belly falling. Feel the breath and belly zipping up the front of the spine. Inhale and return. [*8 times, then proceed through exercise 8 before changing sides.*]

Tip: *Allow space for an orange under the chin and lift from behind the heart, sourcing the head in the core, not the neck. Keep elbows wide, like wings.*

GENTLE VERSION

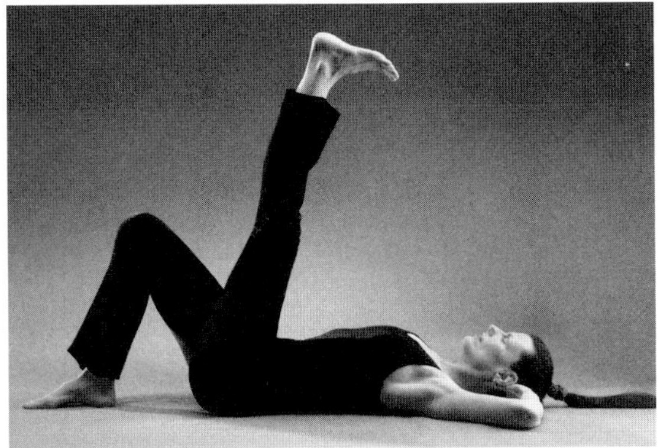

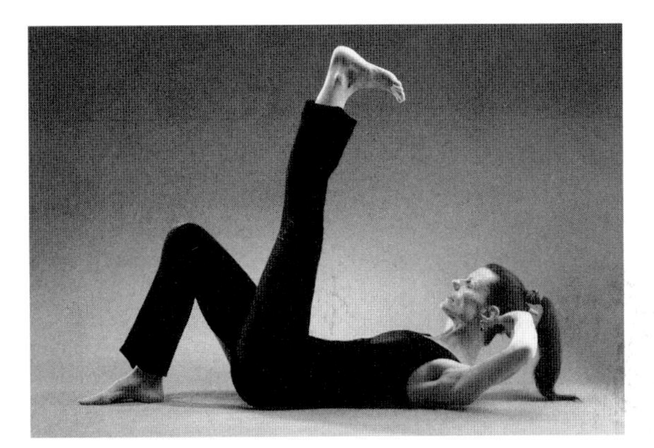

Gentle Version: *Bend your standing leg, plant the foot on the floor, and do the same upper body motion from here.*

8. Open Book/Legover Rock

[for opening hip, spine]

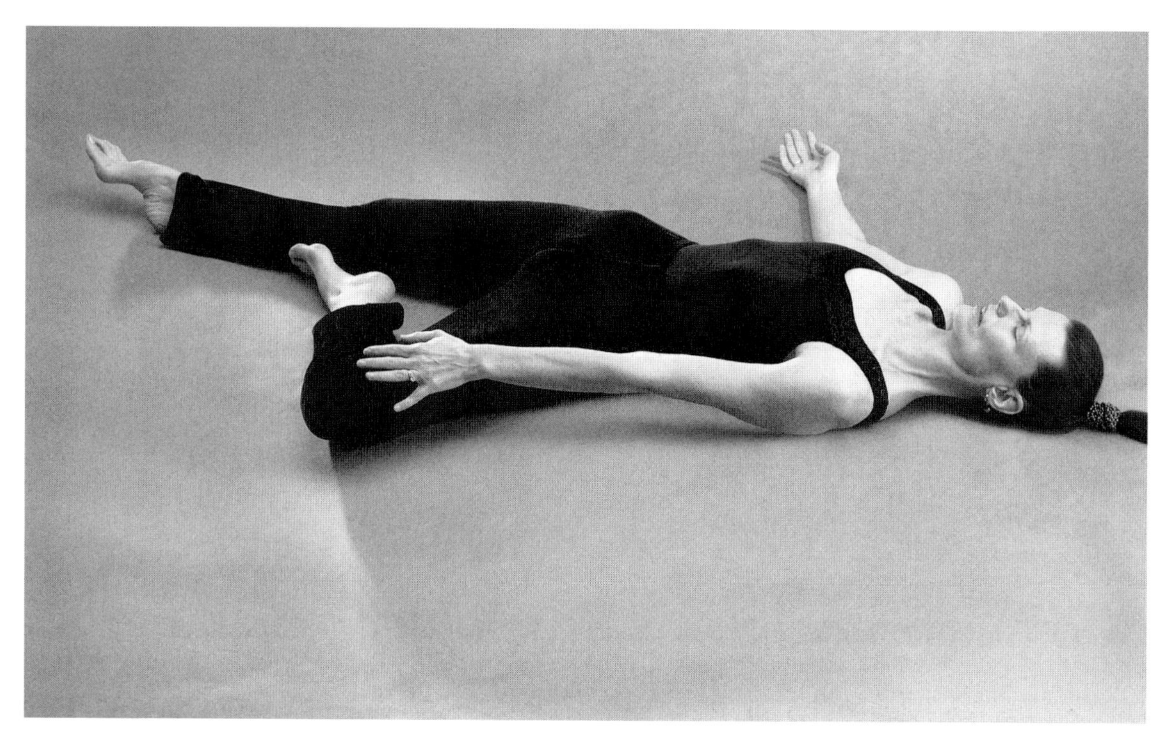

PREPARATION

Return the standing leg long on the floor. Plant the foot of the leg that's been in mid-air on the floor beside the standing leg. Let your knee fall open to the side, like a book that falls open to your favorite poem. Place your hand on the knee and relax.

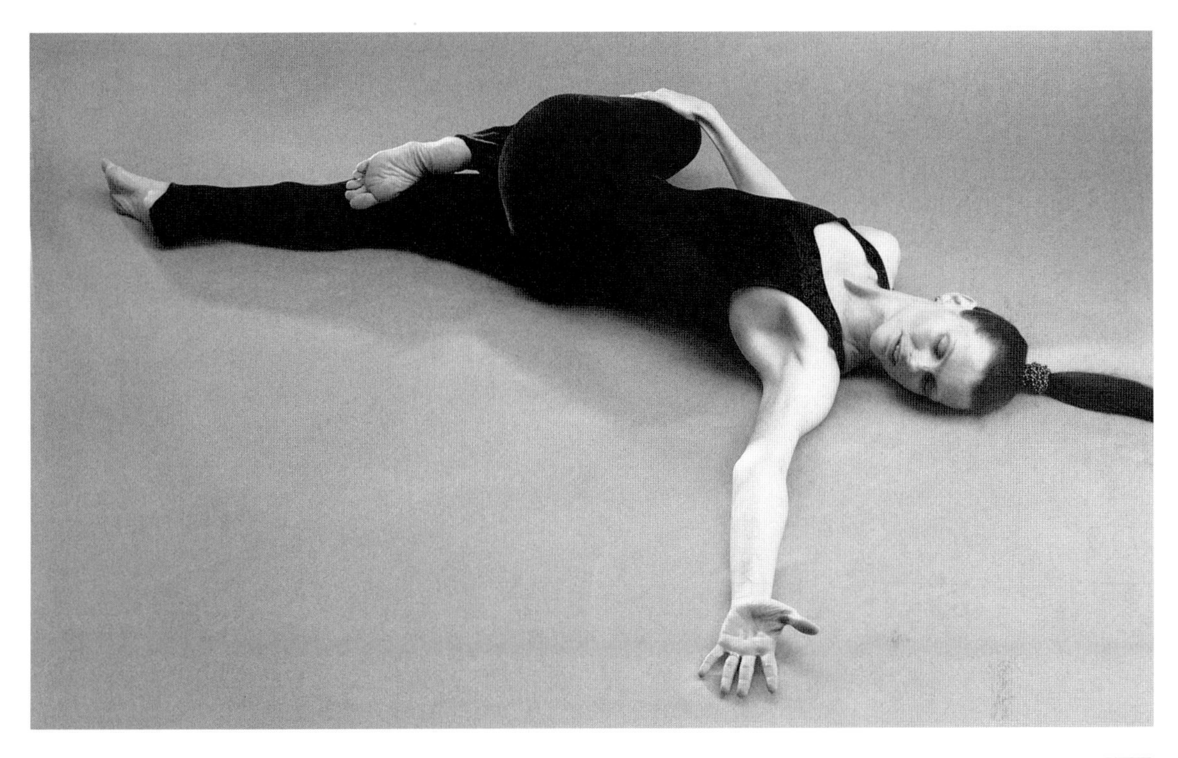

MOTION

Exhale, stepping into the foot and bringing the knee back to center. Fold the knee across your body with the opposite hand, letting your hip come off the floor. Anchor both shoulders on the floor and relax, looking back and stretching into the extended arm.

Rock back and forth several times this way—inhaling to open the knee outward, exhaling to fold across the body and reach back through the outstretched arm. Linger in either position and breathe into the stretch as needed. [*3 rockings, then switch sides and repeat exercises 6, 7, and 8.*]

Tip: *The opposite shoulder (rather than the knee) stays grounded throughout.*

9. Advanced Groaner

[for abdominals, obliques, inner and outer thighs, hips, buttocks]

MIRROR IMAGE

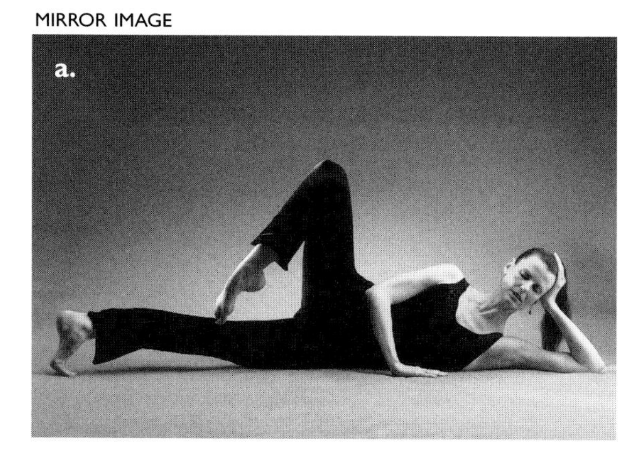

TIP

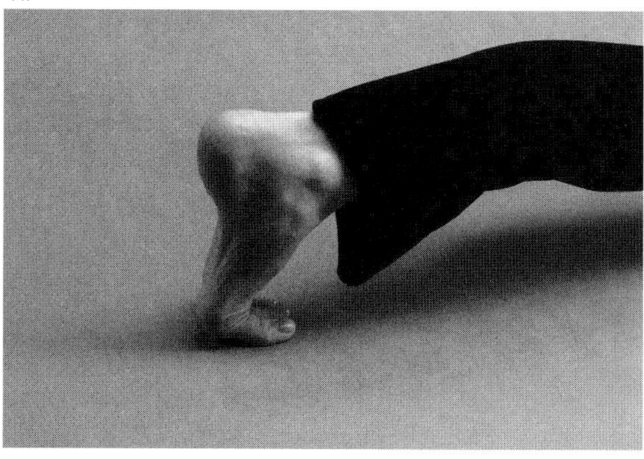

PREPARATION

Centered in the core, roll over to your side (right first) without using your arms or legs. Bend your elbow (right first) and place your head in your hand. The top arm (left first) becomes your "standing" arm, planted in front of your solar plexus. Extend the standing leg (right first) below, at a slight angle in front of the body, and plant the foot one foot-length in front of your hips, resting on the big toe and ball of the foot. The top leg (left first) bends, knee to the sky, toes to the standing knee.

Tip: *Make sure the big toe gets firmly planted so that you can "stand" on this foot. Also, don't let the standing knee bend or touch the floor.*

Gentle Version: *If you find the standing foot position challenging, you're human. Keep striving to get up on the big toe, unless you find it excruciating, in which case, relax the foot on the floor.*

GENTLE VERSION

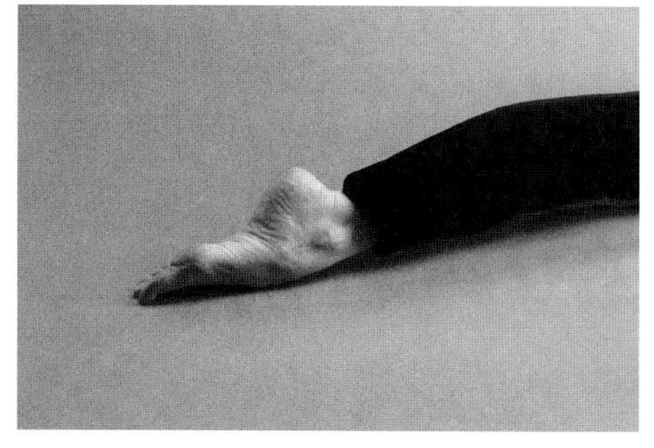

MOTION

Maintain shoulder-over-shoulder and hip-over-hip alignment throughout.

a. Inhale and stabilize your position, top toes to the standing knee, top thigh opened back against the top hip forward. Keep the hips square to the front.

b. Keep inhaling while you lower the top knee parallel to the ground.

c. Exhale and open the top knee back against the top hip, which presses forward.

d. Keep exhaling and extend the leg toward the sky. Hips stay stacked one over the other, like two headlights shining forward on the road in front of you. Inhale and repeat a.–d. [*6 times slow. Before switching sides, do exercise 10 to counteract.*]

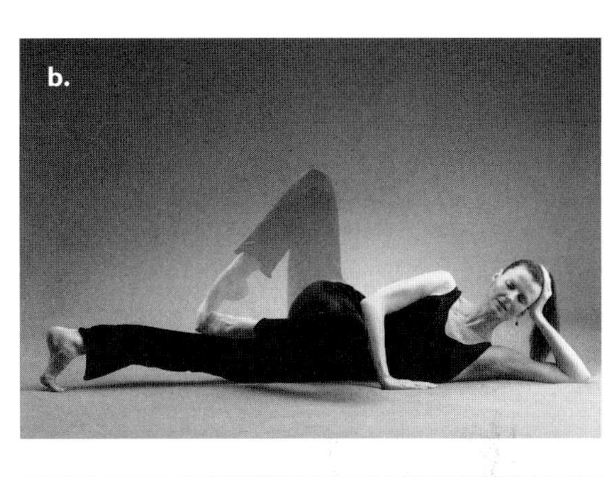

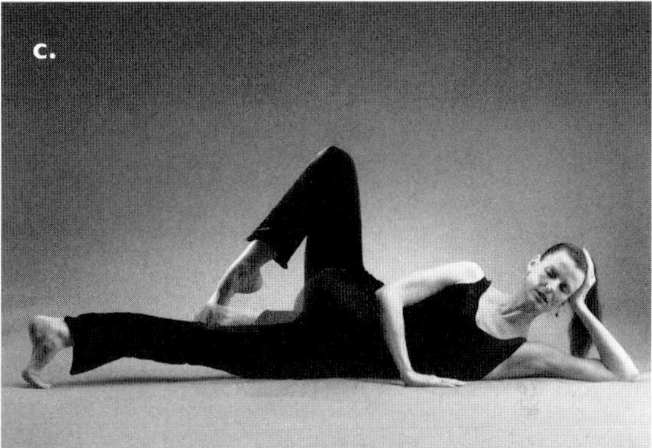

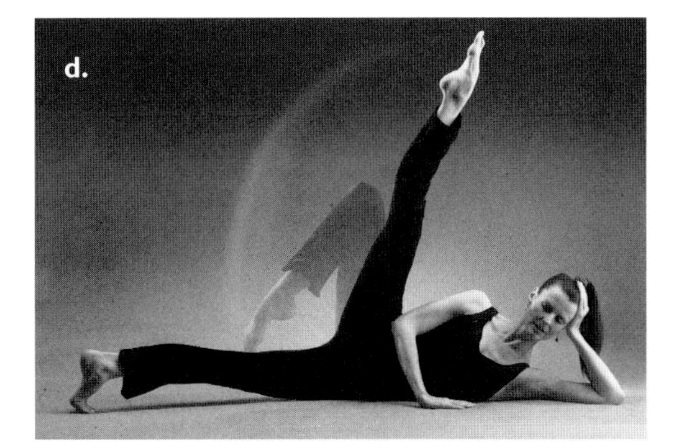

Tip: *Three checkpoints will help you keep your balance. (1) Stay in the core and work from here. (2) Use the standing arm to keep your shoulders square, referring to the core as you push into the hand. (3) Plant the big toe of your standing foot firmly, with the inside of your heel and inner thigh looking forward. This will help maintain your external rotation.*

---

10. Barn Door/Rollover

[for hips, buttocks]

PREPARATION

Bend your standing knee (right first) at a 90-degree angle in front of the hip. Plant the top foot (left first) on the floor above the other knee. Press the top knee open with your top hand. Inhale and breathe directly into the hip and buttock. Exhale and relax. [2 *breaths*]

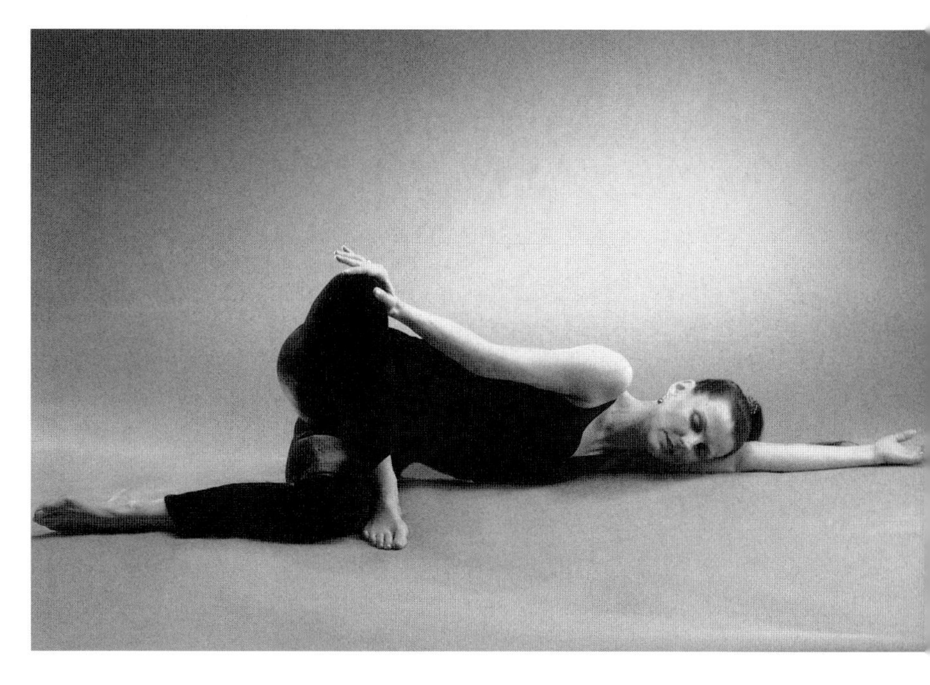

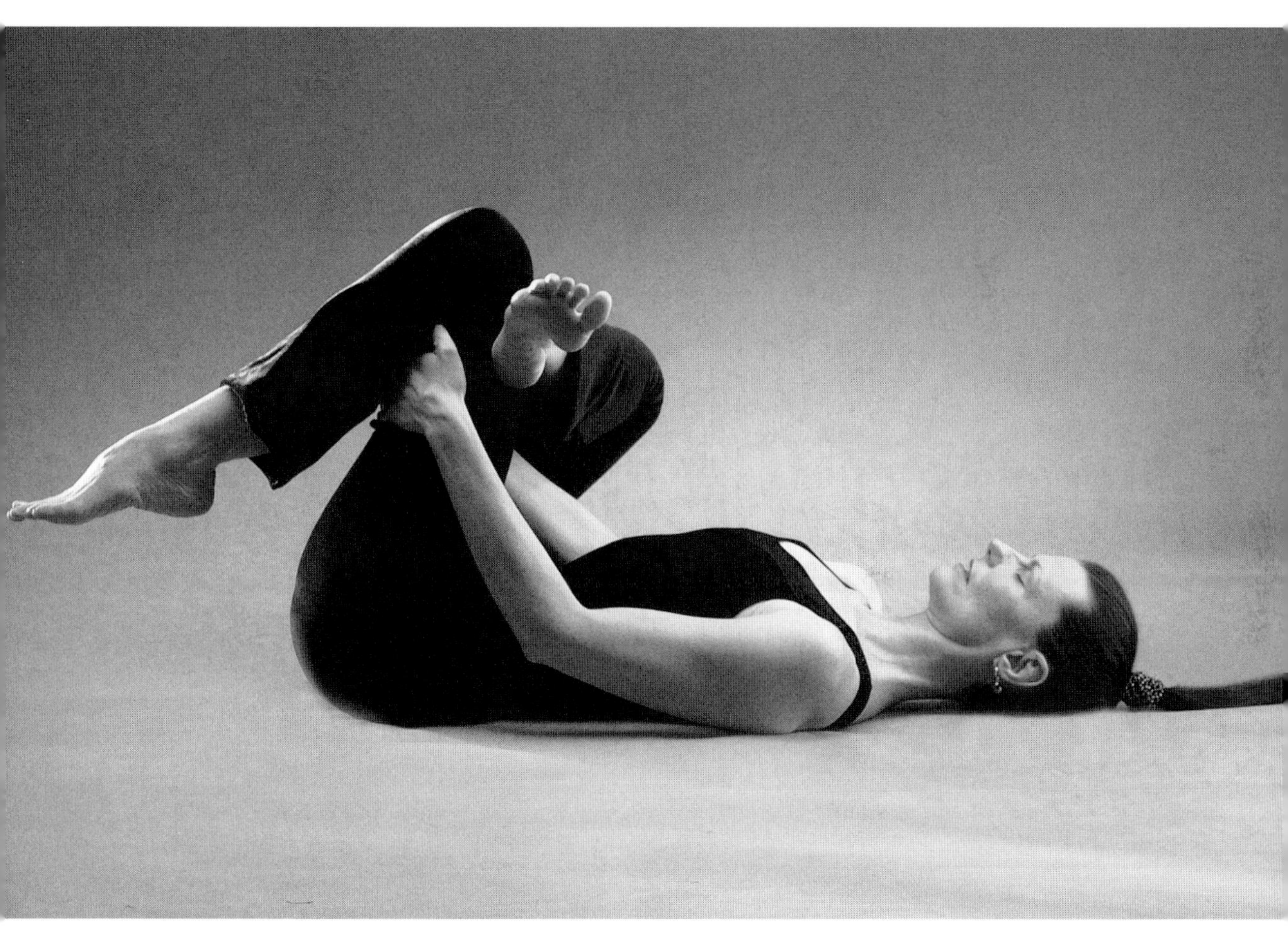

MOTION

Keeping your legs in this position, roll onto your back. Grasp the thigh (right first) that's farther away. Inhale and fill the sensation you feel. Exhale to press the leg into the chest. [*2 breaths, then switch sides and repeat exercises 9 and 10.*]

11. Flatback Diamond

[for hips, spine]

PREPARATION

Using your hands to walk yourself up to a sit, bring the soles of the feet together. Sitting tall, hold your toes and inhale, filling the belly.

Gentle Version: *If sitting with a straight back is difficult in this position, fold or roll up a mat or towel and place it under your hips.*

MOTION

Keeping your spine straight and the front of your torso long, exhale and move forward over the legs. Stay here and inhale, filling the belly, hips, lower back, and wherever else you may feel this stretch. Exhale and lengthen the spine, moving your lower back toward your heels if comfortable, but only as far as you can while keeping the spine straight. [*4 breaths*]

Tip: *Bend from the hips, not the waist. Keep your head in line with the spine by dropping the chin and pointing through the eartips.*

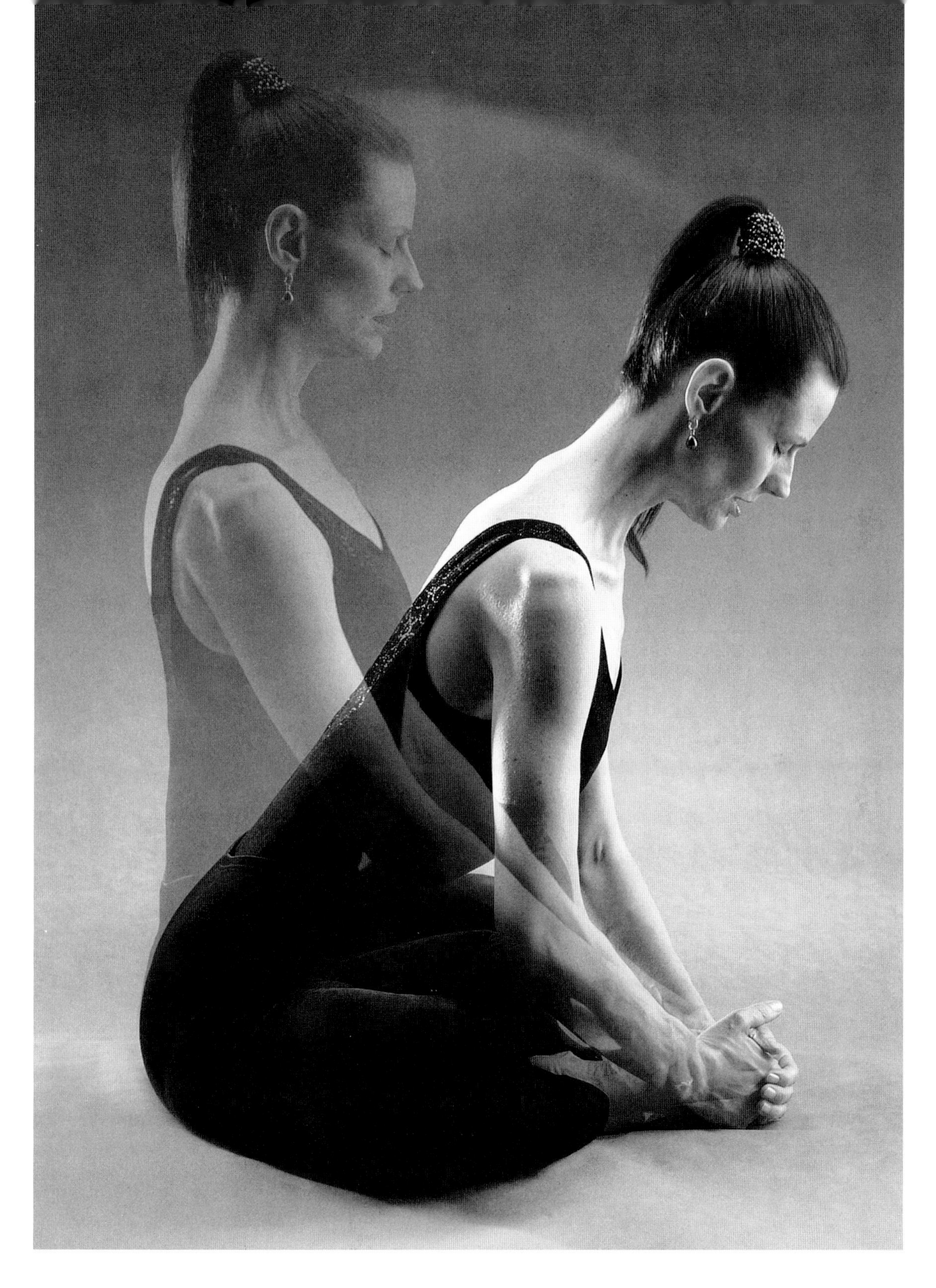

12. Half-Lotus Spiral

[for spine, organs]

PREPARATION

Fold one heel as close to the pubis as comfortable, then fold the other foot in front of the first. Sit tall, pushing the crown out of the belly, and cross your hand (left first) to the knee (right first). Place the free hand behind you, the heel of the hand as close to the tailbone as possible. Inhale, letting the breath fall into the well of the belly.

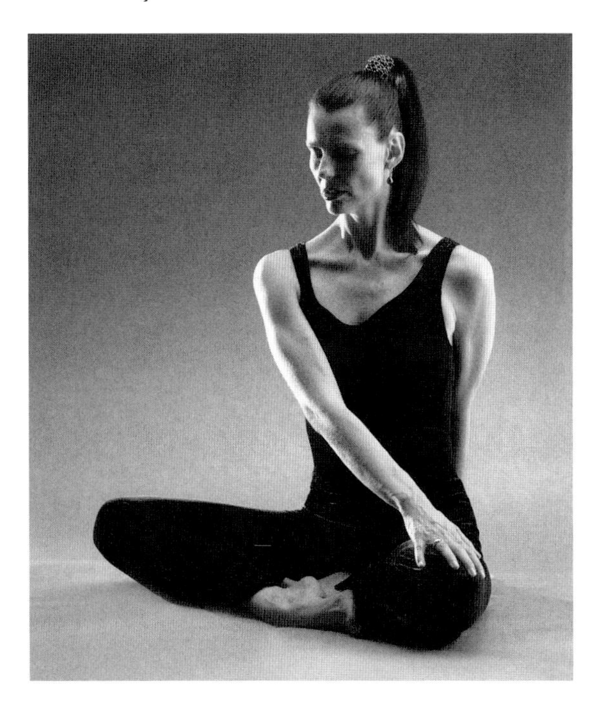

MOTION

Exhale, turning around (right first), looking behind you beyond your shoulder (right first). Inhale, unwinding just enough so that the belly can fill. Exhale and twist a little further, spiraling around your own inner axis. [*3 breaths, then change sides and repeat.*]

Tip: *Do your spiral from the inside out, not from the hands in. Keep shoulders parallel to the earth.*

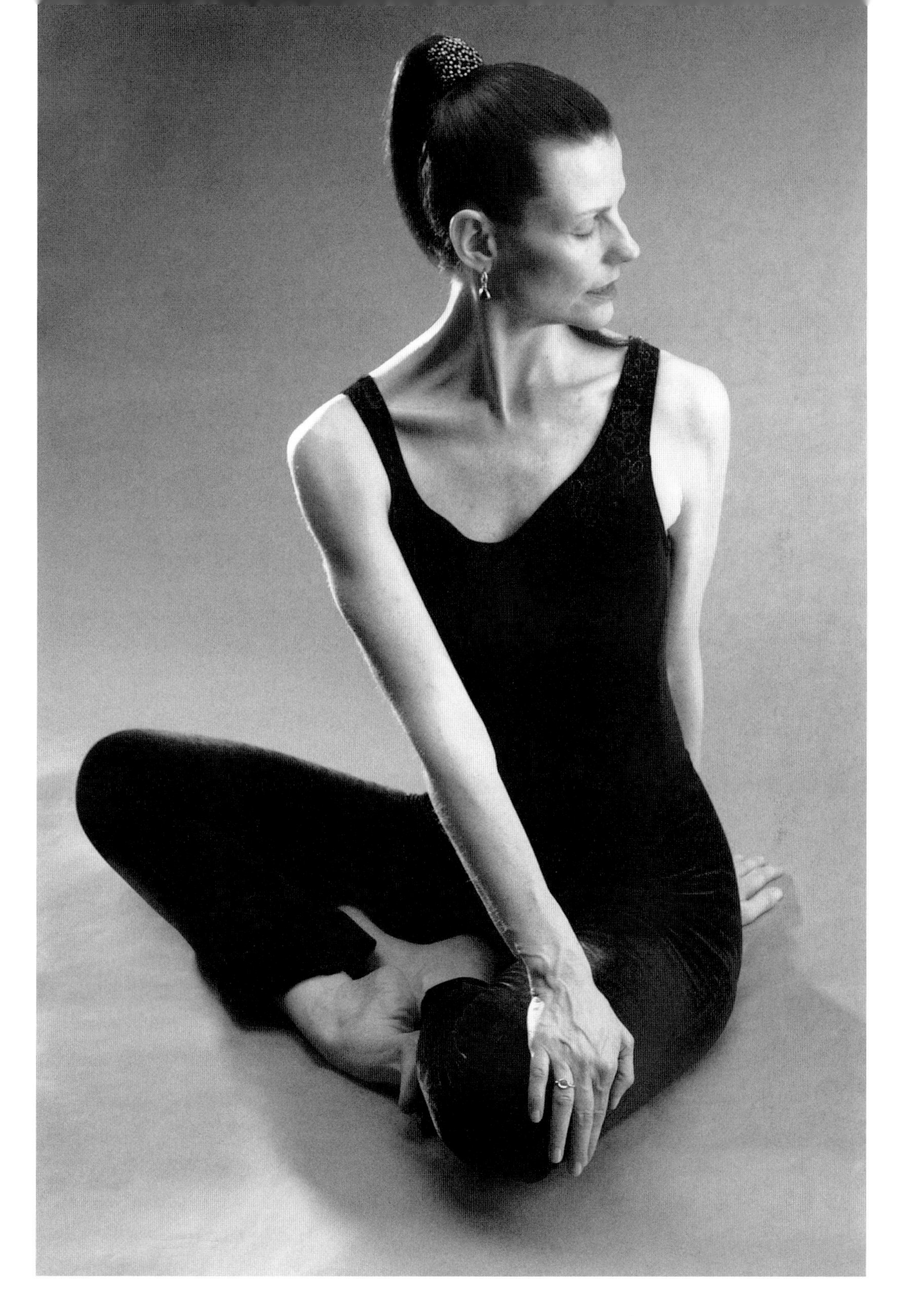

13. Half-Lotus Lateral

[for spine, waist]

PREPARATION

Staying in half-lotus, arms draped to knees, palms up, inhale and let the breath drop through you.

MOTION

Exhale and circle your arm (left first) over the body as you tilt laterally (right first). The standing hand rests on the floor beside the hips. The overhead arm extends into a diagonal slash—a straight line from hip through rib through shoulder through elbow through fingers. Inhale and move through center to the other side. [*6 times, alternating left and right*]

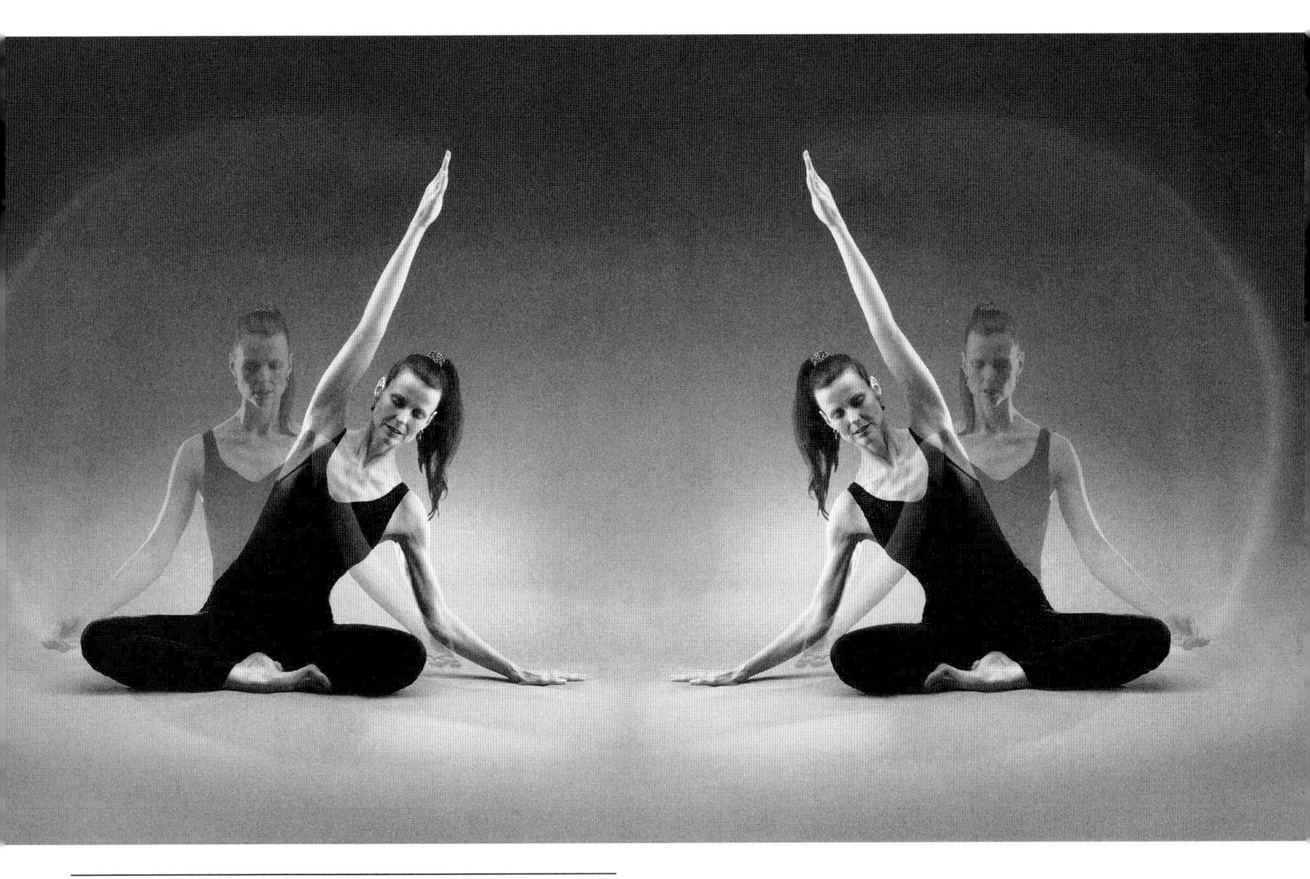

Tip: *Anchor both sitting bones on the floor throughout. Create a straight diagonal line through the arm, shoulder, and hip. (Do not curve at the elbow, rib, or waist.)*

14. Open Fan

[for legs, waist, spine]

PREPARATION

Slide the legs open to 90 degrees, flex the feet, and extend the arms toward your knees. Sitting tall, inhale, letting the breath rain down through you.

MOTION

Exhale, sliding the arm (right first) down the leg (right first), sweeping the top arm overhead and reaching through the fingers, like a paper fan. Inhale and return. [6 *times, alternating left and right*]

Tip: *During the fan sweep, make sure that the top shoulder is aligned directly over the bottom shoulder (not falling forward of it), and that both shoulders are in line over your leg.*

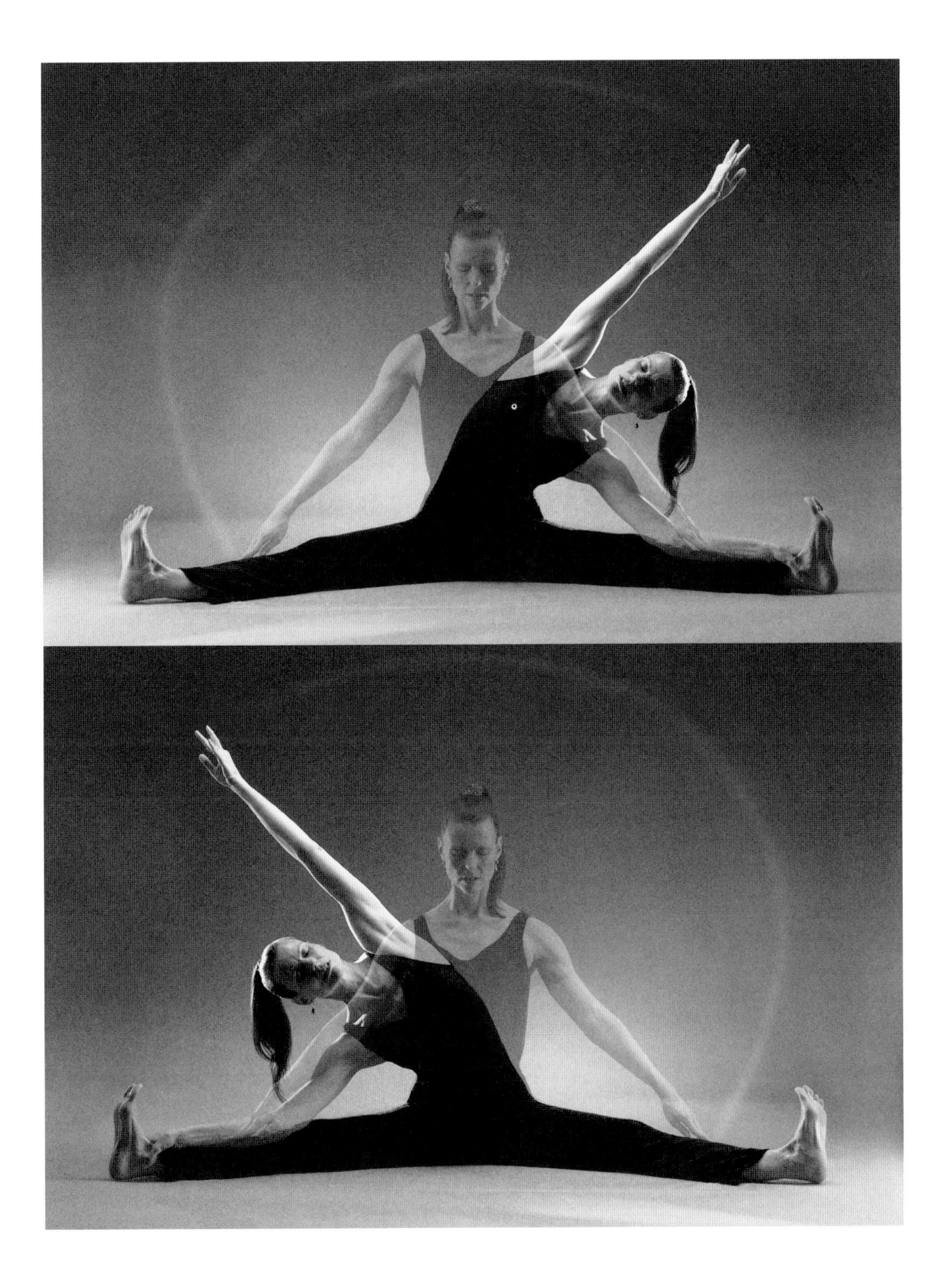

15. Rear Window/Prone Tail Curls

[for lower back, lower abdominals]

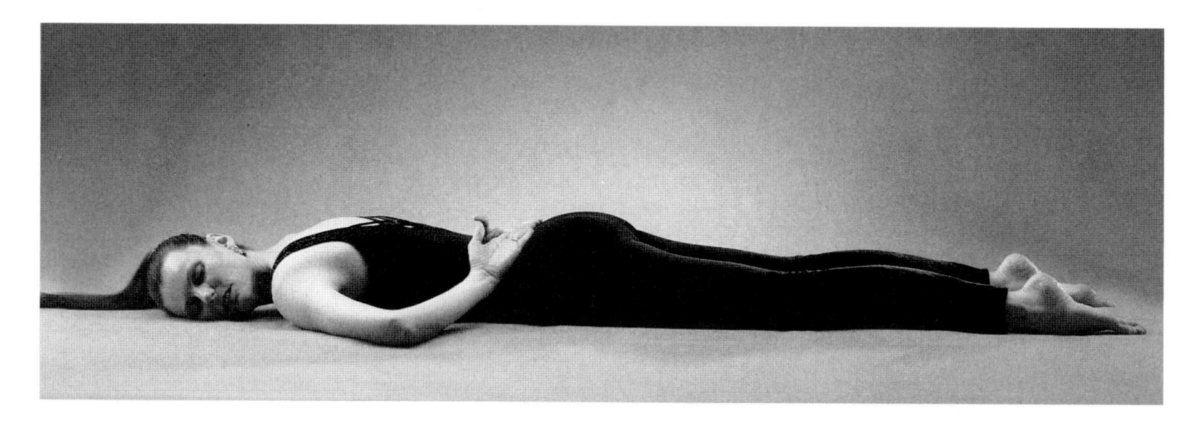

PREPARATION

Sweep the legs to the side and lie down on your belly. Let the legs sprawl hip-width apart in Reverse Corpse Pose. Rest your hands on your lower back below the waist. Close your eyes and breathe through the open window of your lower back, the hands rising and falling in response. [*4 breaths*]

Gentle Version: *If your back doesn't like this position, roll up your mat or towel and place it under your belly. If your hands aren't happy on the lower back, fold them under your brow or place them at your sides.*

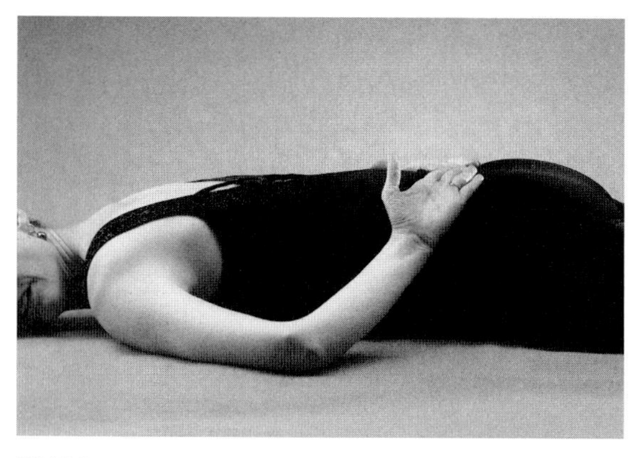

INHALE

EXHALE

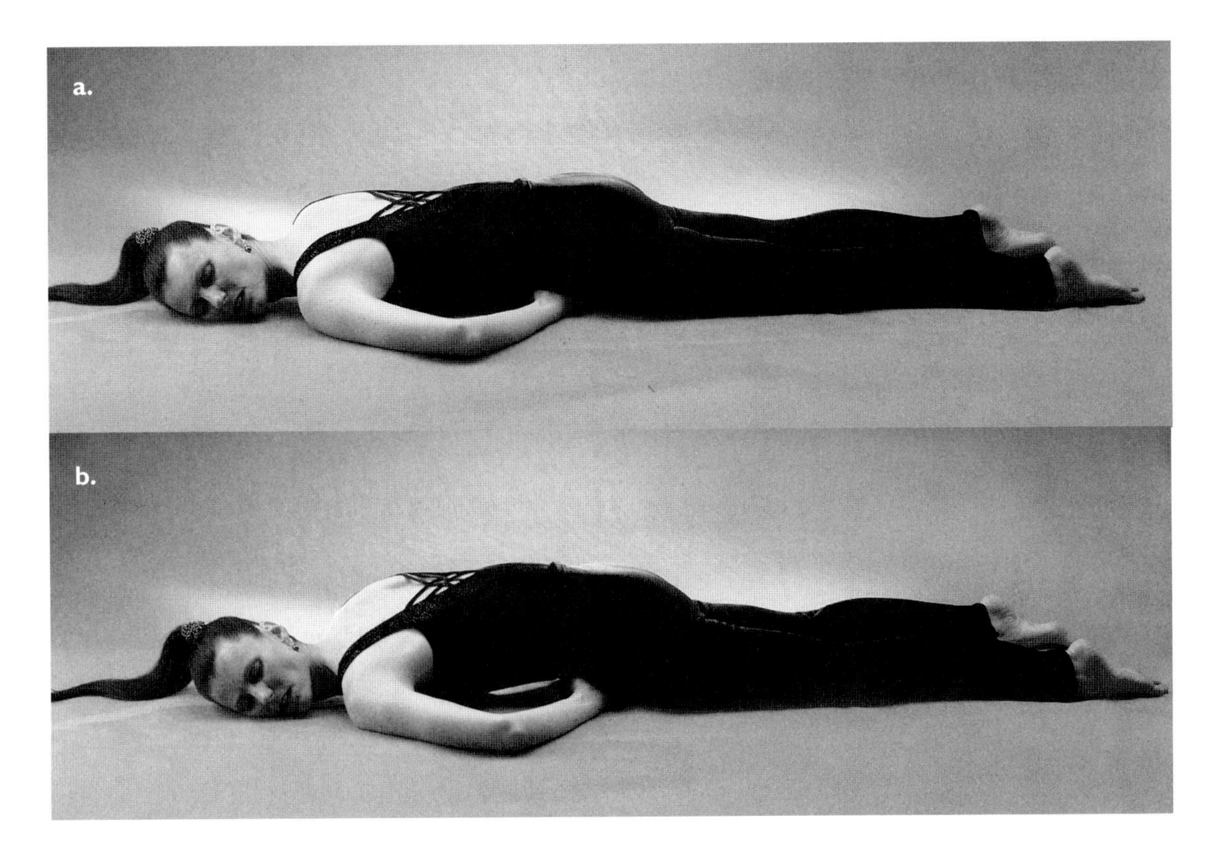

MOTION

a. Relocate your hands under the low tummy and inhale.

b. As you exhale, curl the tailbone under (without clenching the buttocks). Your belly will naturally scoop inward as it follows the exhalation along the front of the spine, ultimately creating space between the belly and hands. Inhale and return. [*8 times*]

Tip: *This is a wholly abdominal exercise, so don't let the buttocks block the way by clenching. If done properly and slowly, Prone Tail Curl is exquisitely excruciating. During the exhalation, the back of the waist is high, the tail sloping downward.*

16. Tail Plunge

[for lower back, core]

PREPARATION

Still in Reverse Corpse Pose, clasp the hands behind the waist and inhale.

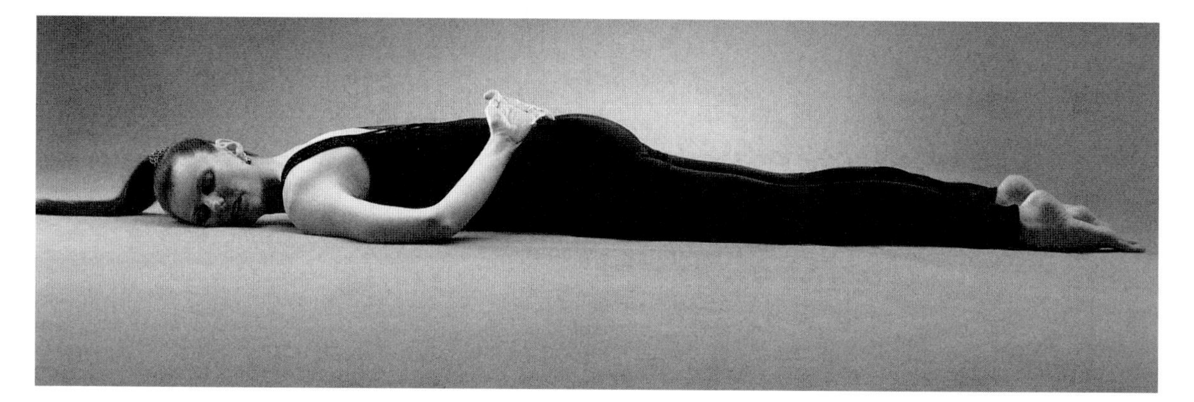

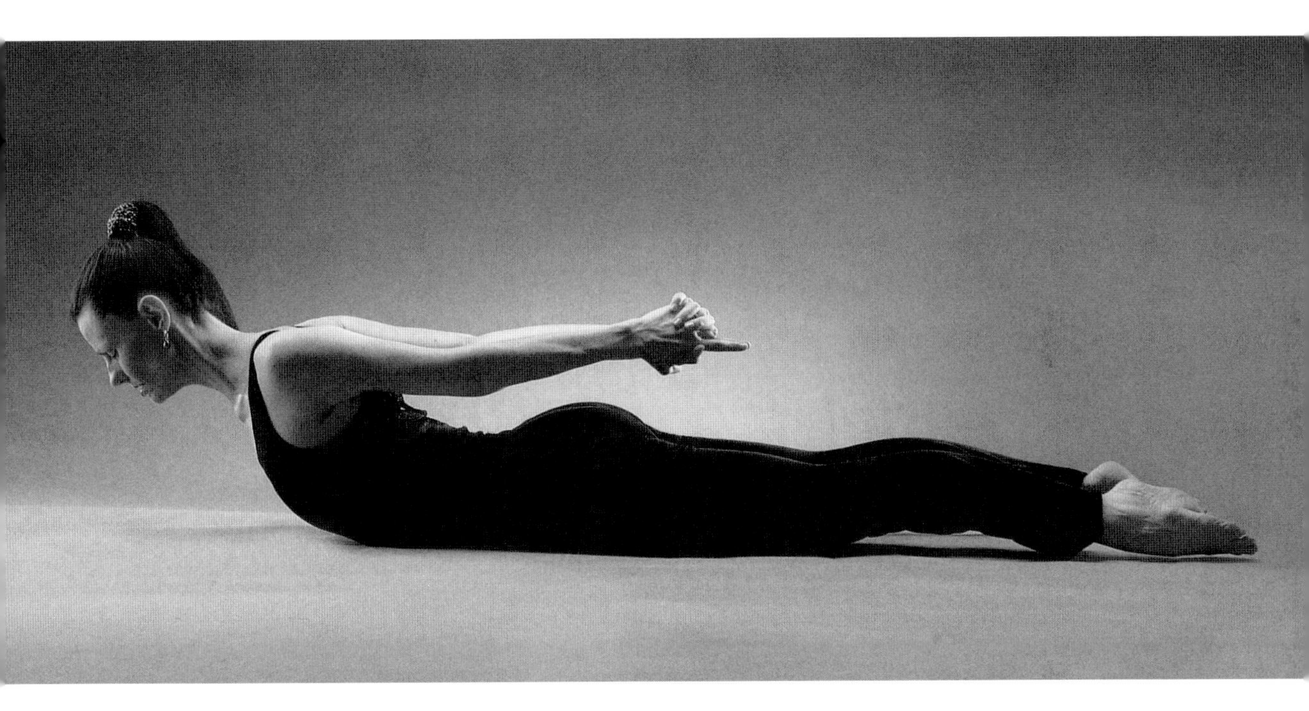

MOTION

Exhale, plunging the hands down beyond the tailbone (pointing index fingers if you like), lifting your upper body off the floor. Inhale and slowly return. [*4 times*]

Tip: *Keep the back of your neck long. Support from the core.*

GENTLE VERSION

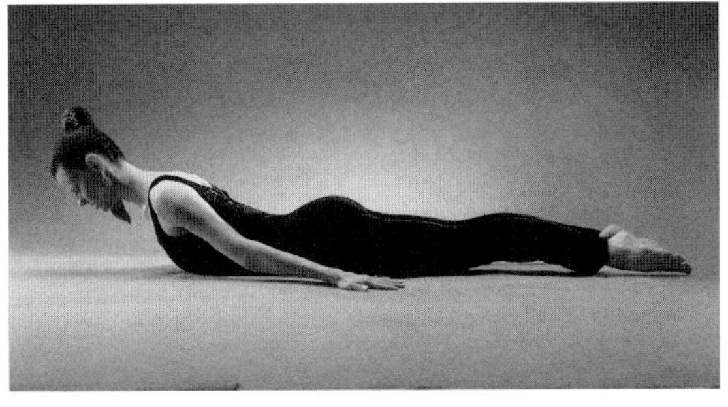

Gentle Version: *If holding your hands behind your back is uncomfortable, place the hands at your sides, palms down.*

17. Half-Cobra

[for spine, core]

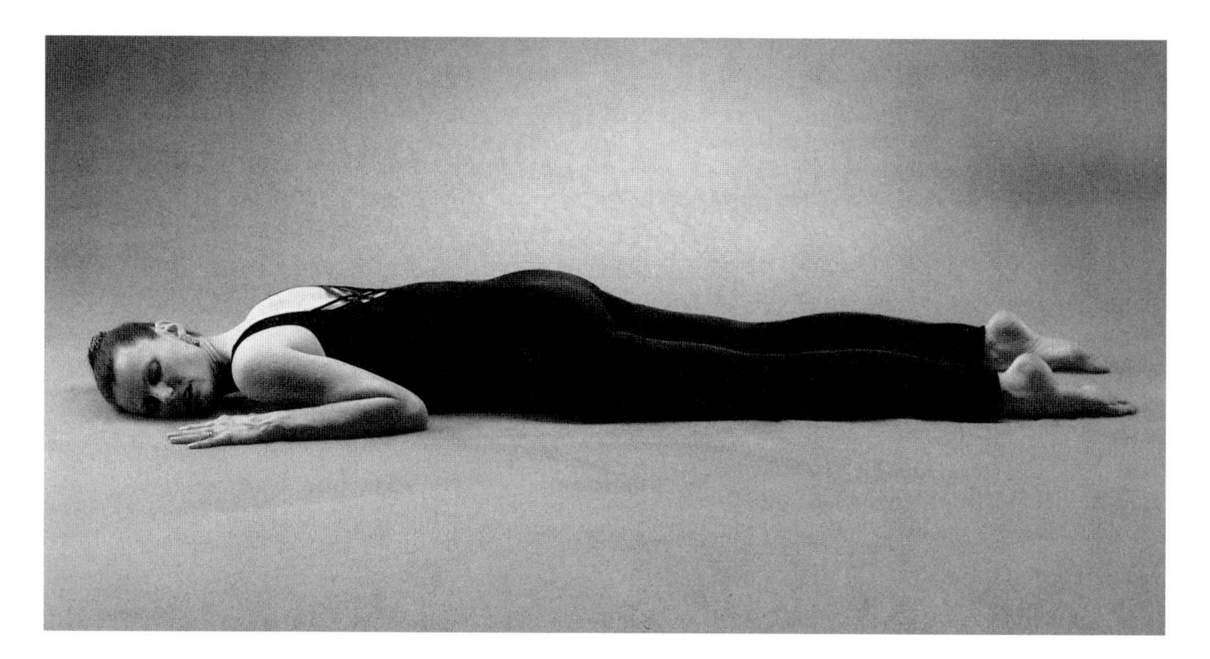

PREPARATION

Still prone, place the hands palms down beneath your shoulders, fingers spread, elbows on the floor beside ribs. Inhale and fill the lower back.

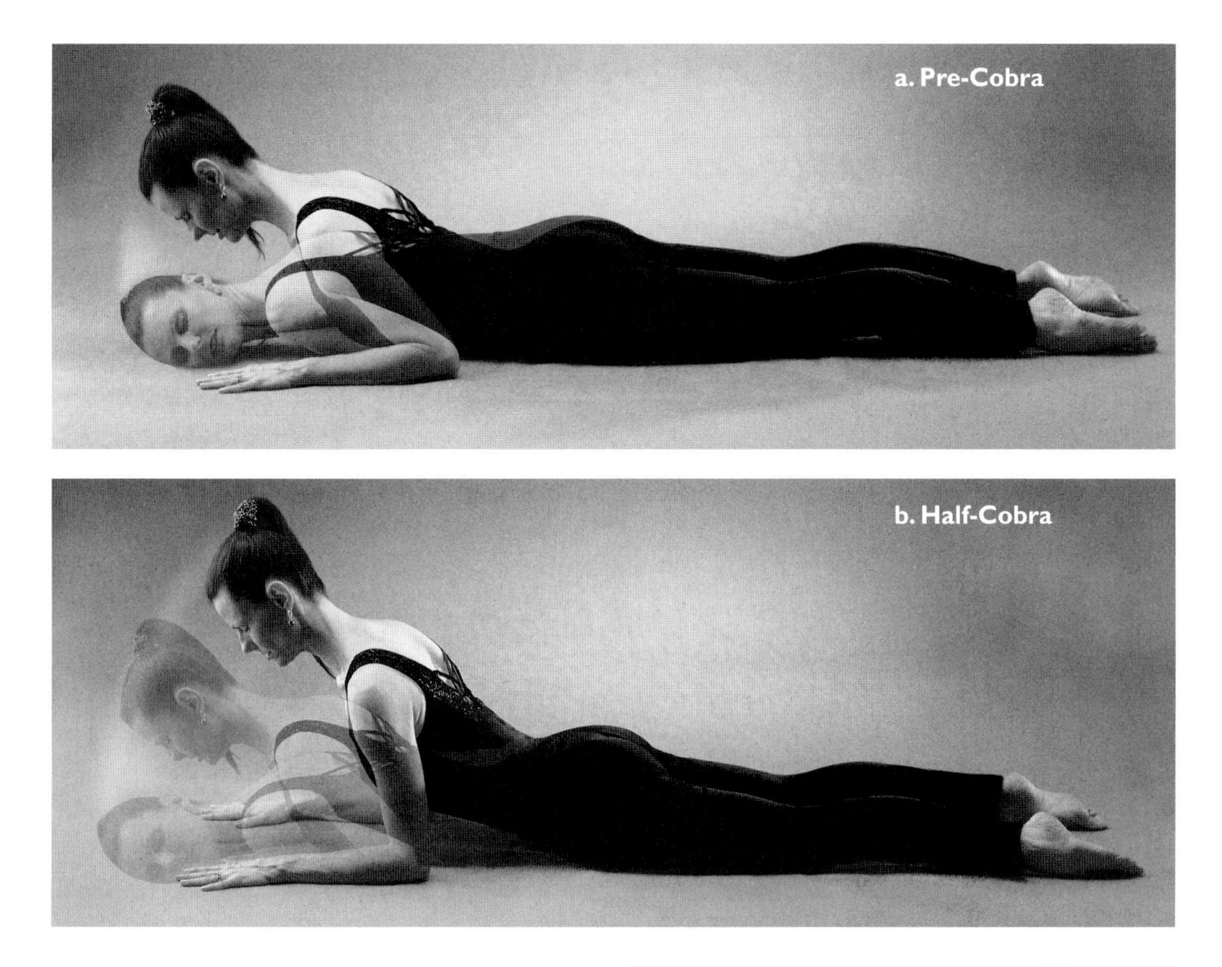

MOTION

a. Exhale and do Pre-Cobra, first *extending* the spine, then *ascending*—lifting the upper body without yet using the arms. Inhale and gently lower, filling the lumbar chamber. [3 *times*]

b. Exhale, lifting the upper body as far as the core muscles will take you without using the arms. At your peak, blend a little weight into the forearms and push up higher, keeping elbows on the floor and shoulders down. Inhale and lower, working your way down. [3 *times*]

Tip: *Keep the transition between using the core muscles and the arm muscles smooth, almost imperceptible.*

18. Cat/Table Pushups/Baby Pose Cycle

[for spine, inner thighs, abdominals, hamstrings, biceps, triceps, pectorals]

PREPARATION

This series cycles through three motions from the beginner workout. Coming up to all fours, place the hands directly beneath the shoulders, knees beneath hips, hip-width apart. Spread your fingers and push down through your arms. Lift the head and tail and inhale, filling the belly.

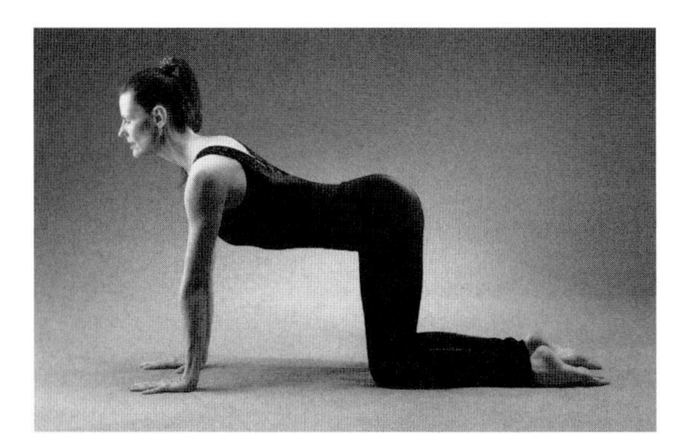

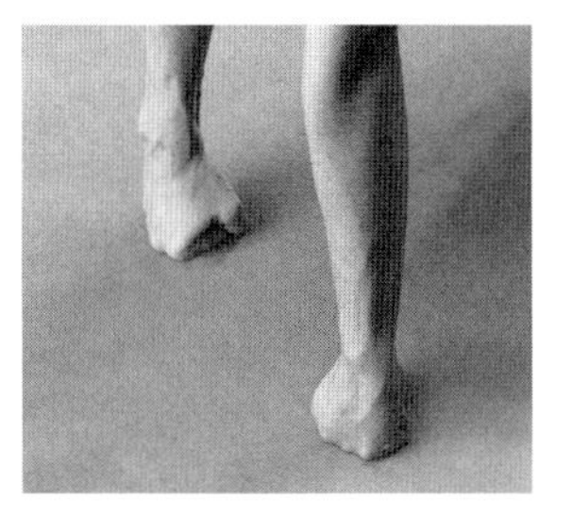

Gentle Version: *If this position hurts your wrists, get up on your fists for both (a) and (b).*

MOTION

a. *Cat:* Exhale and curl the tailbone, undulating slowly through the spine from the bottom up. If you like, count your vertebrae as you roll through each one, until at the end of this fluid motion the head falls and the back of your heart rises even higher. Inhale and return.

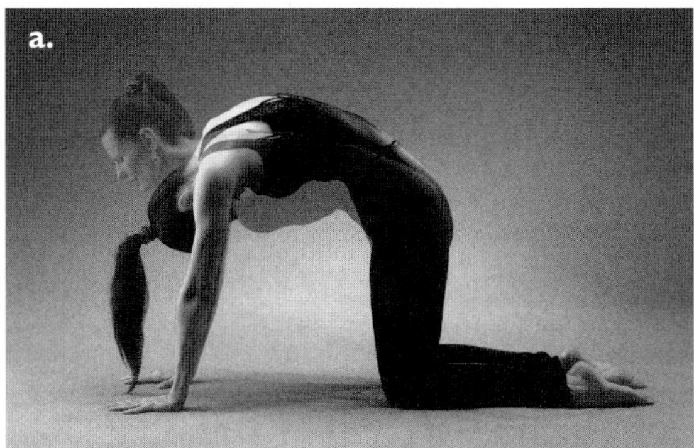

b. *Table Pushups:* Flatten your back. Inhale, bending the arms and lowering your upper body toward the floor. Exhale and straighten. [*4 times, then 16 pulses*]

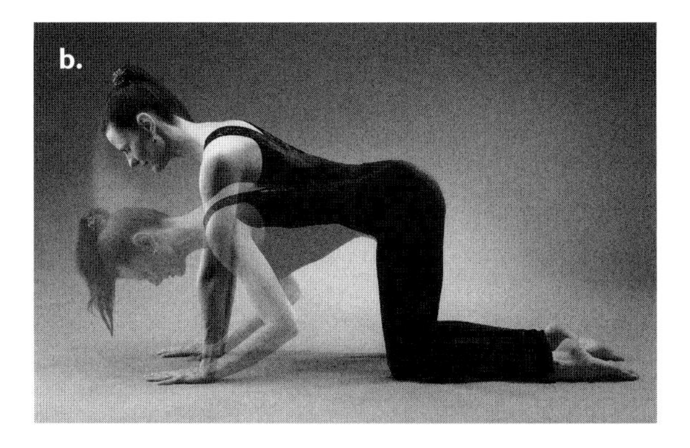

Tip: *Keep the back straight, head in line with spine (not dropped toward floor).*

c. *Baby Pose:* Sit back on your heels and rest. Legs are hip-width apart so that your belly and chest can fall between the thighs. Place your head comfortably on your brow or cheek, letting the arms stream out in front of you or at your sides. Rest here, breathing into different parts of your back that call for attention, feeling them billow out like a pillowcase filling with wind. [*about 45 seconds*]

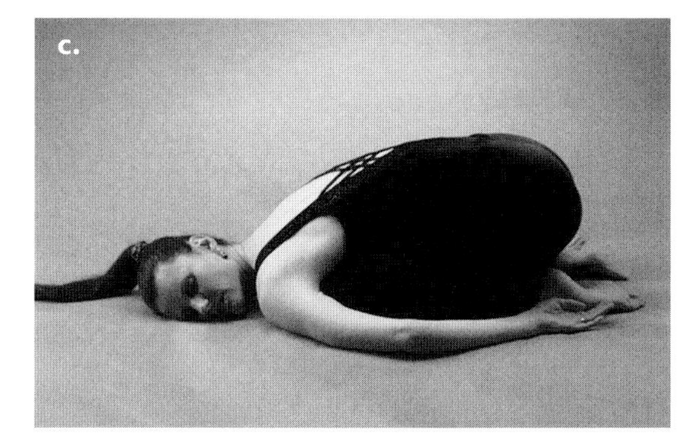

d. Cycle through the sequence again, from Cat through Table Pushups (this time vary the pushups by placing hands together under the heart center, the tips of thumbs and forefingers meeting in a triangle), then finish in Baby Pose.

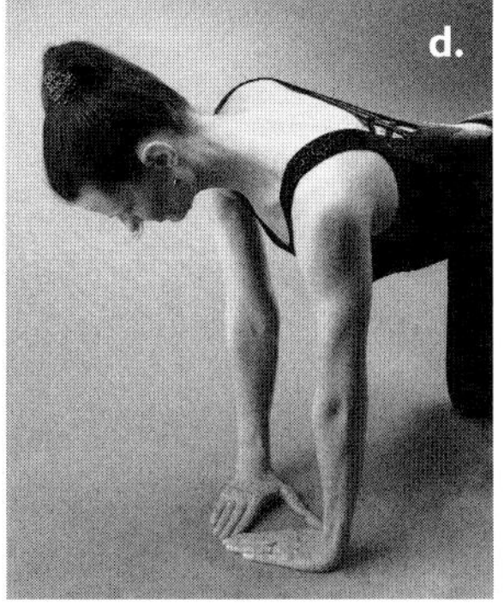

BABY POSE GENTLE VERSIONS

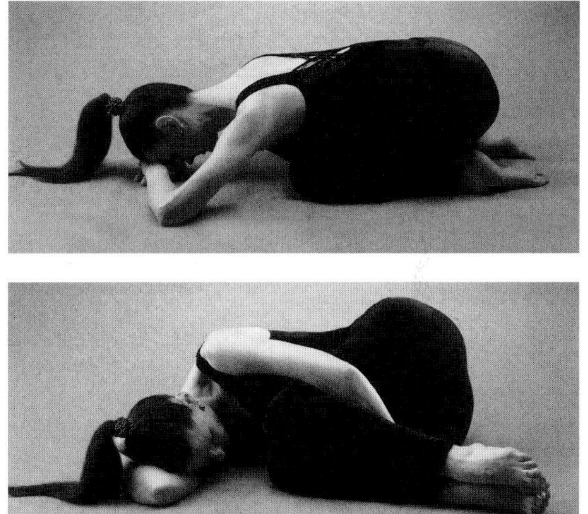

Baby Pose Gentle Versions: *Place your hands (or fists) under your brow and ease the hips back down toward the heels. If your knees are an issue, turn on your side in fetal position and rest, breathing into the back and any tension you discover.*

19. Intermediate Tail Curls/Wing Lifts

[for abdominals]

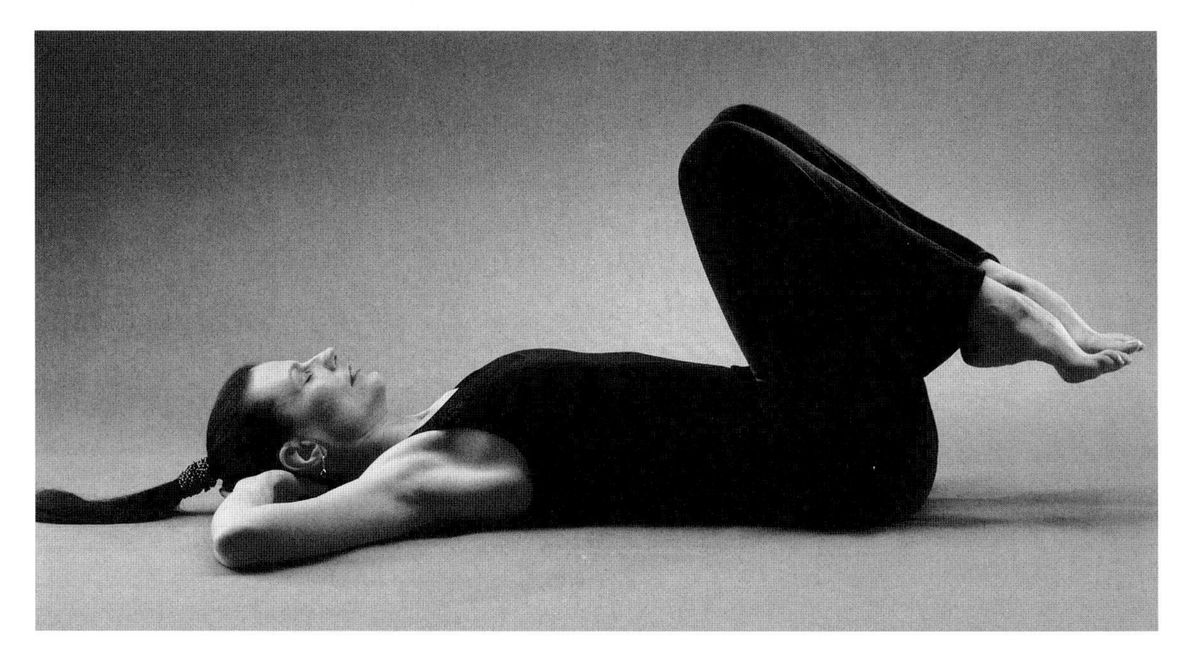

PREPARATION

Without using your arms, roll over on your back. Now bend the knees to the chest and lace your fingers behind your head. Inhale, filling the belly.

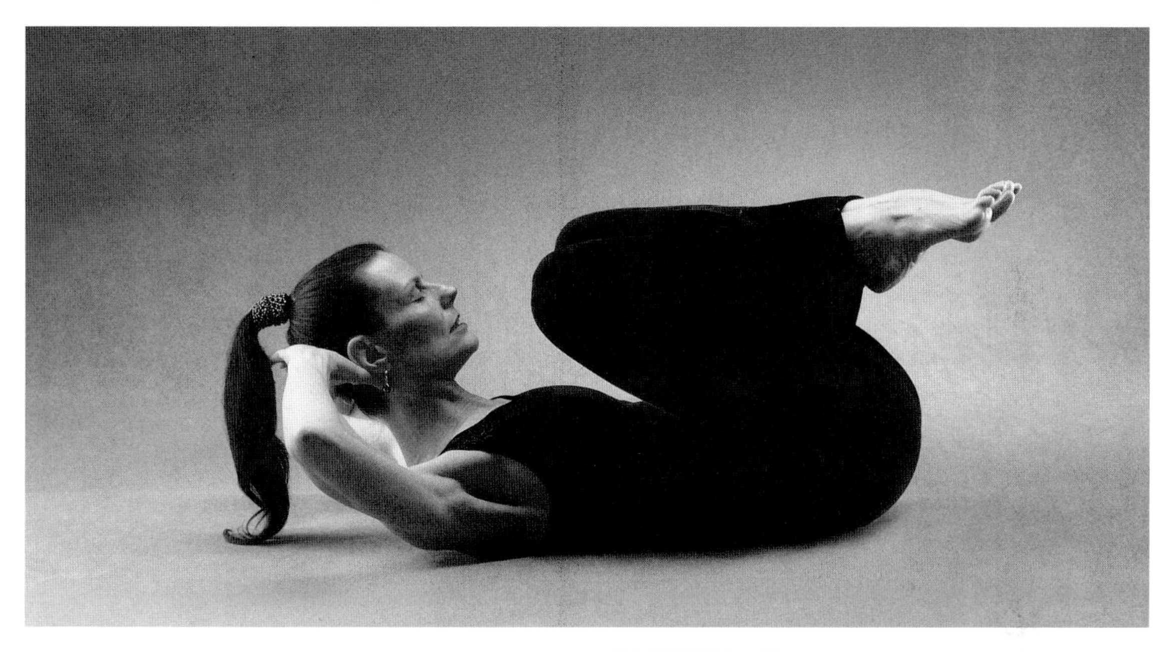

MOTION

Exhale as you (1) curl the tail, (2) empty the belly, and (3) lift the wings (shoulder blades) off the floor, riding the flow of the exhalation through the heart. Inhale and unroll. [*4 times slow, then 16–32 pulses*]

Tip: *Curl the tail to the head, not vice versa. Keep your elbows wide and lift the upper body from behind the heart. Each time the wings rise, the belly must fall in response to the exhalation.*

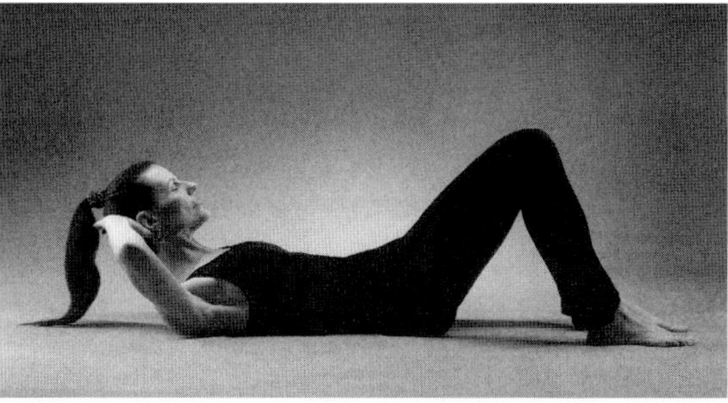

Gentle Version: *If this hurts your back, or if you simply prefer, plant the feet hip-width apart on the floor and do the same motion from here.*

20. Corpse Pose

[for relaxation, realignment, rejuvenation]

To finish, return to where you began. Let the legs stream out, hip-width apart, arms 45 degrees from the sides of your body. How different this place feels from when you first visited! Feel how the body has opened, how clear and spacious a place it is becoming.

Inhale, breathing through the heart down along the extending pathway. Exhale and return along the spine, feeling the natural fusion of the abdominals and the wind. Travel the path for as long as you wish, gently gliding into the space between breaths, a space that begins to expand as you relax more deeply.

After a while, let go of the breath and simply bask in the shimmering energy that radiates through you. Let this energy permeate every cell and organ, beaming through every pore like a star that shines out in all directions. This is your natural state, a depth of grace and peace that underlies everything you are and everything you do. Remain here as long as you like.

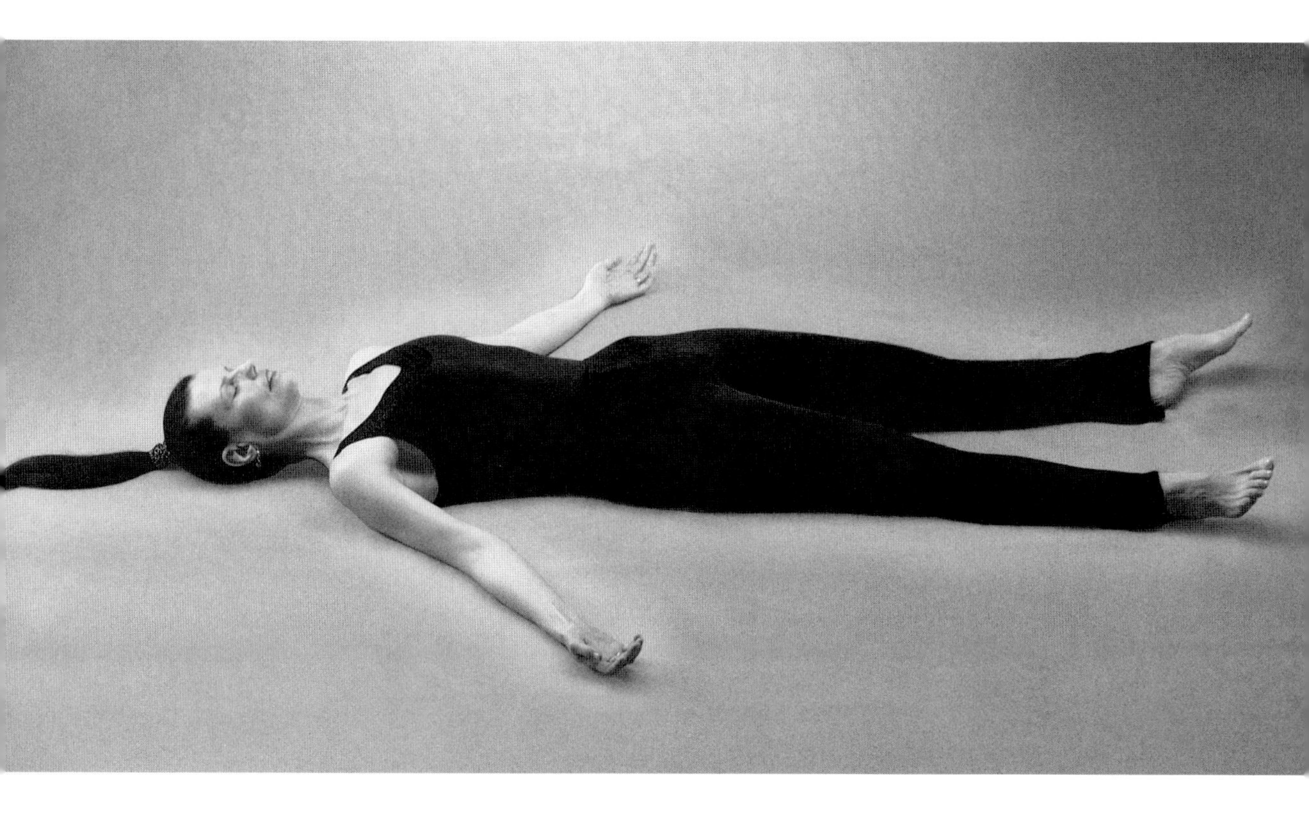

Yoganetics for Intermediates: Flow Chart

Condensed Photo-Map of the Workout

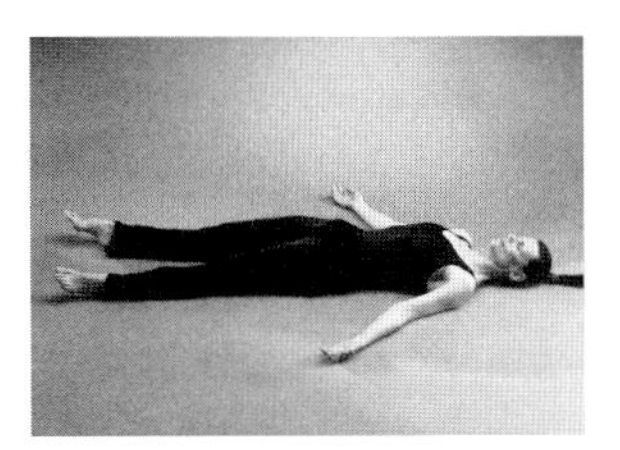

1. Corpse Pose (p. 90) [*5-minute voyage, 8 path breaths*]

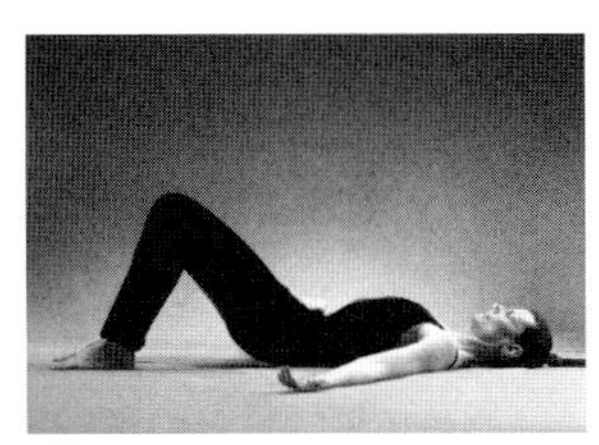

2. Tail Curls (p. 92) [*8 times*]

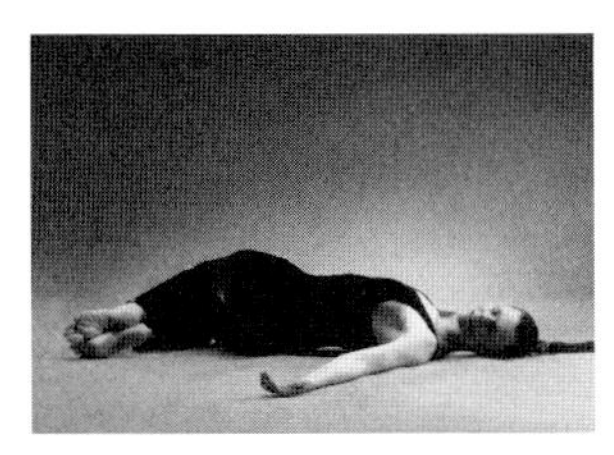

3. Double Legovers (p. 94) [*6 times, alternating left and right*]

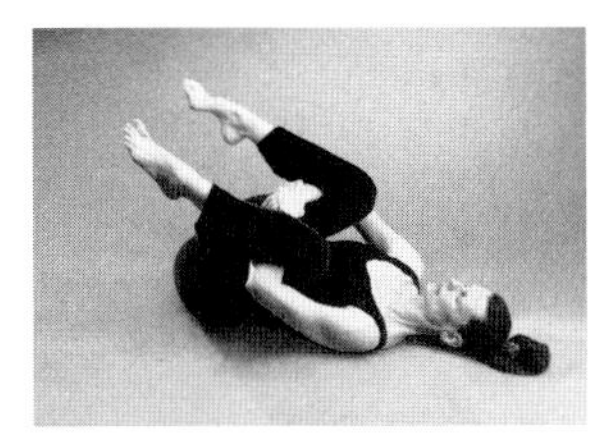

4. Double Leg Press (p. 96) [*4 breaths*]

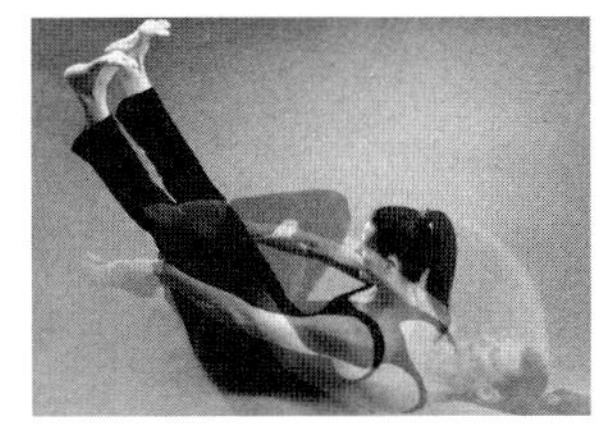

5. Double Leg Push (p. 98) [*2 parallel, 2 turned in, 2 turned out*]

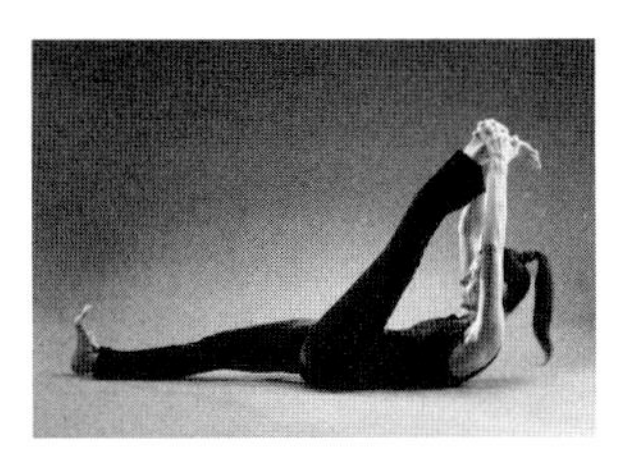

6. Separated Leg Push (p.100) [*2 basic, 2 with hold, 2 with dive*]

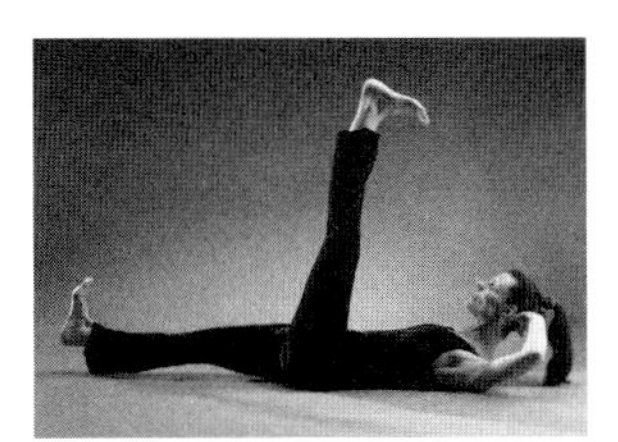

7. Yoga Zip-ups (p.102) [*8 times each side*]

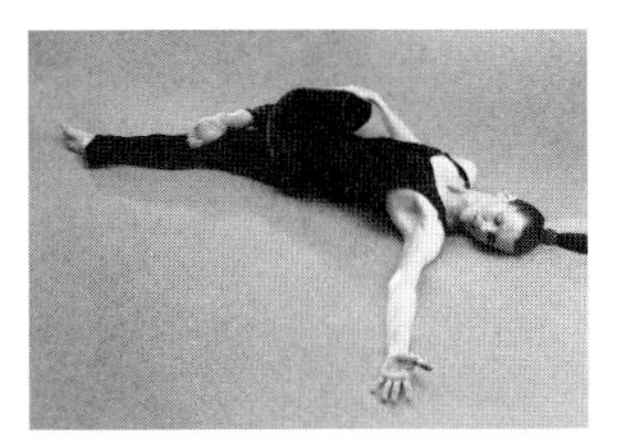

8. Open Book/Legover Rock (p.104) [*3 rockings*]

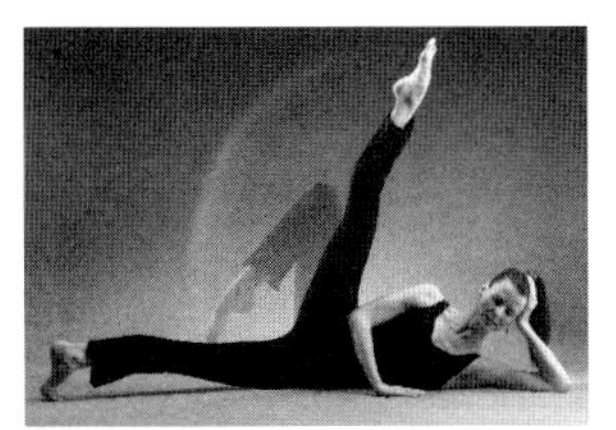

9. Advanced Groaner (p.106) [*6 times*]

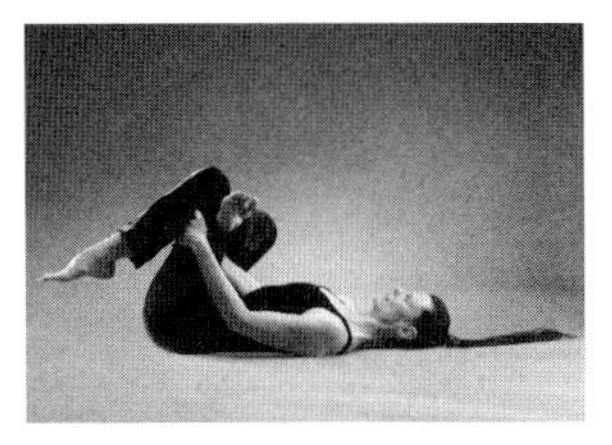

10. Barn Door/Rollover (p.108) [*2 breaths each position*]

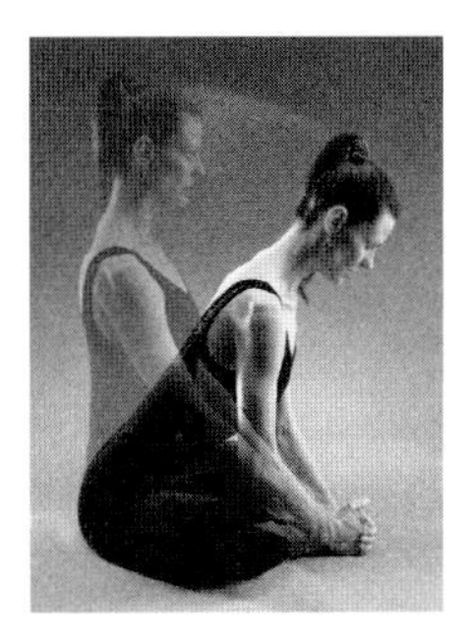

11. Flatback Diamond (p.110) [*4 breaths*]

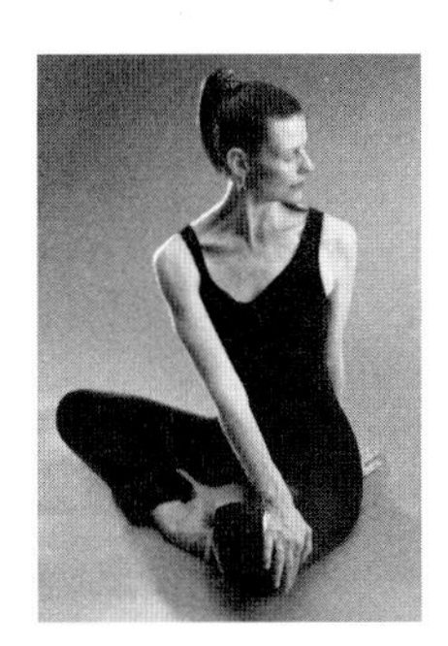

12. Half-Lotus Spiral (p.112) [*3 breaths each side*]

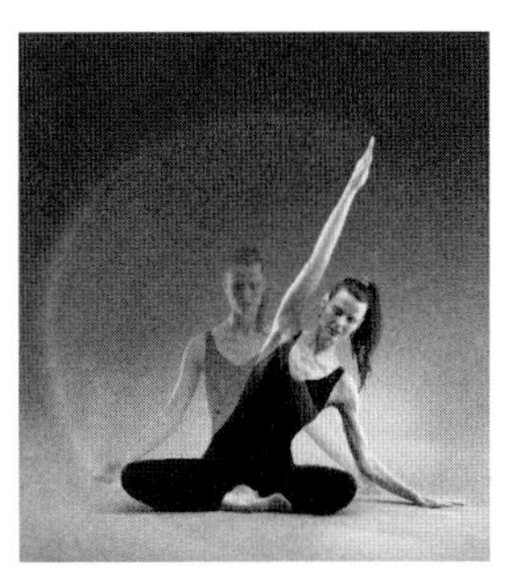

13. Half-Lotus Lateral (p.114) [*6 times, alternating left and right*]

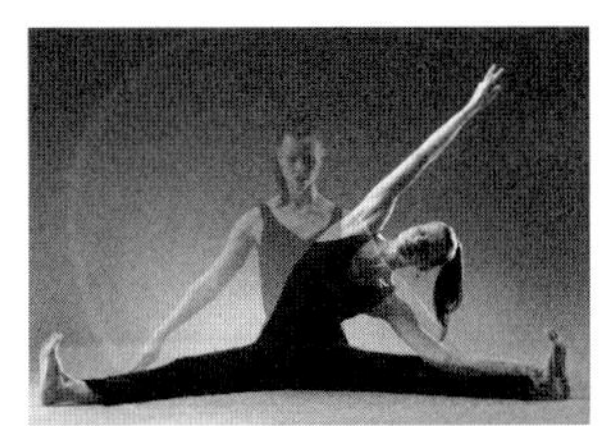

14. Open Fan (p.116) [*6 times, alternating left and right*]

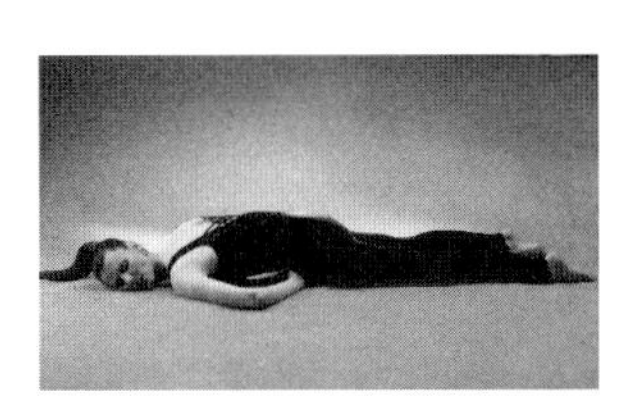

15. Rear Window/ Prone Tail Curls (p.118) [*4 breaths, 8 curls*]

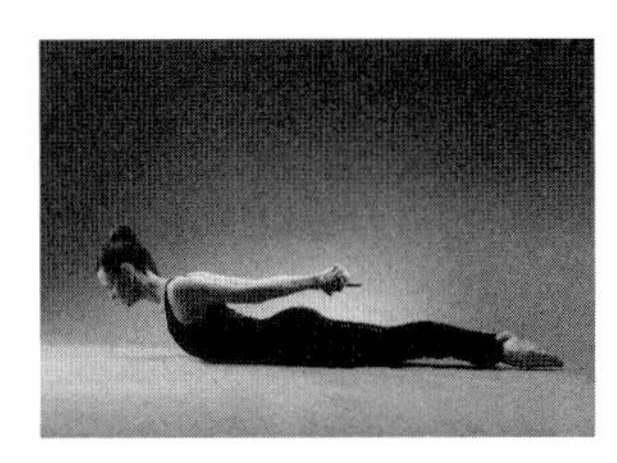

16. Tail Plunge (p.120) [*4 times*]

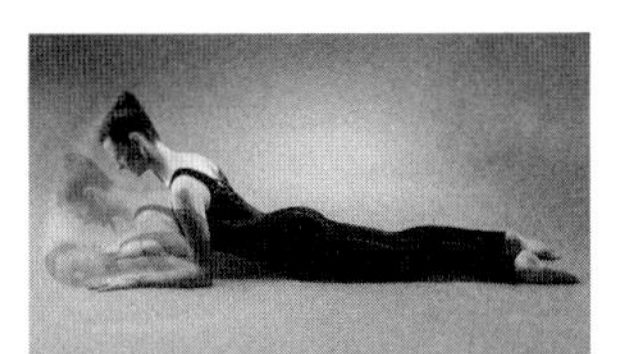

17. Half-Cobra (p.122) [*3 times Pre-Cobra, 3 times Half-Cobra*]

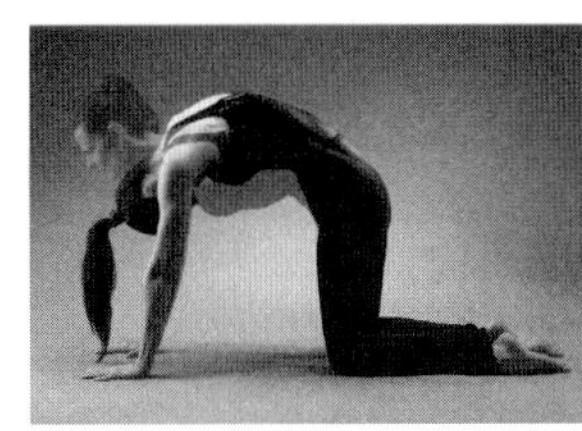

18. Cat/Table Pushups/ Baby Pose Cycle (p.124) [*Cat: 1 time; Pushups: 4 times, 16 pulses; Baby Pose: 45 seconds; cycle through twice*]

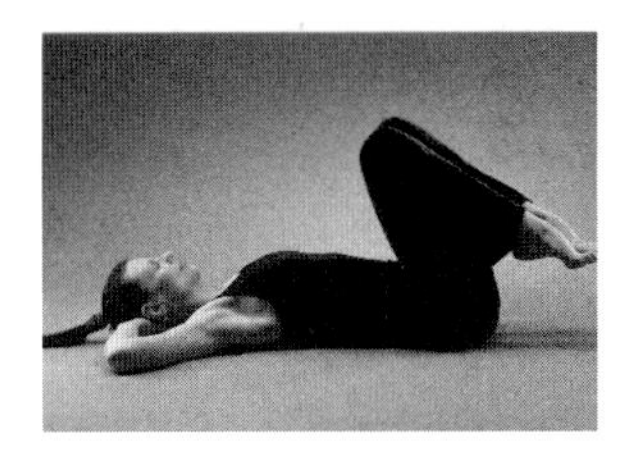

19. Tail Curls/Wing Lifts (p.126) [*4 times, 16–32 pulses*]

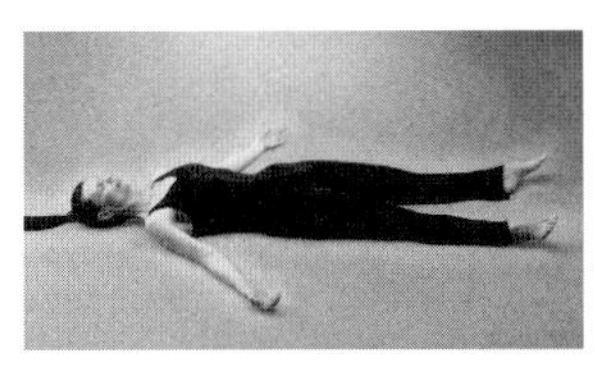

20. Corpse Pose (p.128) [*meditation*]

Part Three

Beyond the Mat

Eight

Unconscious Exercise

Then the big gate swung slowly open, and they all passed through and found themselves in a high arched room, the walls of which glistened with countless emeralds.

L. FRANK BAUM, *THE WONDERFUL WIZARD OF OZ*

Our mission is not to practice yoga for an hour several times a week, but to transform all of life into yoga. Once we rise from the mat, our bodies go along for the ride through the rest of our day, moment by moment, hour after hour. To realize fully our experience of living in the body, we must translate what we are learning in our practice to the "unconscious exercise" that fills our lives: the sitting, standing, walking, climbing, reaching, bending, and lifting that cumulatively determine the body's welfare.

In these final three chapters, we extend yoga beyond the mat into every aspect of daily life. But before we train in the new, we must train out the old. Physical re-education begins with unlearning whatever doesn't serve us—all the years of accumulated idiosyncrasies that are not only habitual but harmful. We may not even be aware of these habits—from the merest frown to a clenching in the stomach—but they dam the flow of energy and drain the life force.

We start with awareness, by turning on lights where there was darkness and taking a look around. Stress is the perfect invitation to do just that. Let's look at what happens in the microcosm of a single hour. Specifically, notice what the body does during the next sixty minutes when it encounters a little stress.

Experiment: **The next time you hear a sudden sound, or glimpse an awful headline, or get cut off in traffic, or feel any other kind of stress, become aware of your body. What is happening inside you? Are there places where you physically deposit your tension?**

It's always interesting to discover the sites we favor, the secret pockets of tension into which we have been making regular deposits all our life. Some people are jaw clenchers, while others dig trenches between their eyebrows. Many, especially those who work at a desk, use the neck and shoulders as repositories for tension. Others prefer the lower back.

Some people internalize tension by going even deeper—organ deep. Many favor the stomach and tend toward digestive disorders. Others get headaches. Wherever your main repository is, it is a place you have returned to countless times, whether or not you are aware of your visits.

As you become familiar with your preferences, you'll find you have a primary repository as well as several secondary ones. My primary repository is my lumbar spine, with my brow and jaw in secondary roles. These three are entwined in my body as a "stress reflex." As we begin to undo the primary, the secondaries will also respond.

People's choices are fascinating—as rich and varied as the lives that created them. To discover your primary and secondary repositories, do the following experiment. The results may surprise you.

Experiment: **Make a Geography-of-Tension Map. Use a sheet of paper to draw an outline of your body's front and back sides. Keep your map handy—perhaps beside you at your desk—and then spy on yourself for a week. Every time you feel yourself tense up, put a stroke on the page corresponding to the place you feel it. At the end of the week, tally up your strokes. The site with the most strokes is your primary repository; the others are secondaries.**

This exercise is empowering because once you discover your own secret pockets, you can turn them inside out and expose them to light. Awareness is everything.

Experiment: Close your eyes and visit your primary repository. Visualize a path from the heart center extending directly into this place. Now inhale, traveling the path and filling its exact shape and size with wind. Feel it expand and open as you inhale. Exhale, and imagine it deflating. Breathe here for one minute.

How does this feel? Did you notice a shift as your awareness and breath entered through the locked door of your tension?

It cannot be said enough: If you are depositing tension in these spots amid uncomfortable situations in life, you are probably doing the same thing in uncomfortable positions in yoga. Your practice is a microcosm of your life and provides a regular opportunity to reverse negative patterns. Every time you do Yoganetics, monitor the sites where tension has kept you from feeling at home.

We must guard the castle of the body vigilantly from the invasion of tension—not by locking down but by opening every door and window, then ensuring that they *remain* open. By unlocking the body, we allow ourselves access to the core of our being, where the deeper, essential work takes place.

The Great American Pastime

Once we're conscious of our areas of tension, it's time to extend our awareness into a larger domain, into an activity so pervasive it cuts across race, religion, class, age, and gender. We may think we lead diverse lives, but every day millions of us are performing the very same action, whether we're answering the phone, writing a letter, or reading a book. You're probably doing it right now—as am I.

We're a nation of sitters. As soon as we get out of bed, we sit down to breakfast. We crunch ourselves into cars that funnel us out into the world, then sink behind a desk until we sit down to lunch. Then back to the desk, car, and home again, where we hover over supper, then pour the body into its favorite chair until bedtime.

With all the practice we get, you'd think we'd be experts. But sitting has led to an epidemic of back pain, a syndrome affecting 80 percent of Americans.

"Sitting is terrible," says Dr. Arthur White, an orthopedic surgeon and former president of the North American Spine Society. "In societies that don't have chairs, people sleep on the ground, and when they meet on the trail, they squat down and get their weight off the back of their discs. Ground-dwelling cultures don't have significant back pain," he observed after visiting Africa and Polynesia.

"No one should sit all day," agrees Dr. Eric Rasmussen, a chiropractic orthopedist in Prairie Village, Kansas. "A lot of people do—and they end up with a herniated disc, which they associate with lifting something the wrong way. But that's not the case. People can sit there and waste away. Posture is a big part of that."

The good news: We don't have to squat on the ground to transform sitting into a form of exercise. Research shows that sitting properly actually *burns twice the calories* as slouching. The benefits extend beyond the physical into mental and emotional realms. While taking a much dreaded drive home for the holidays, one student noticed that sitting well "reduced the stress and helped me to become more alert and energetic. The trip was the best I've had."

Hunchers, Slinkers, and Crossers

If you're interested in raising your metabolism and energy level naturally, don't move—not, at least, until you've done the following experiment. In learning to sit erect, your first task is to discover what kind of sitter you already are.

Experiment: **Close your eyes and notice how you're sitting. The posture you've chosen probably isn't the most efficient, but it's familiar—a pose you have returned to again and again. Now, let's sink even deeper into it. Imagine that it's the end of a long day and you're very tired. How do you sit when you are exhausted?**

People generally fall into three categories: the Slinkers, the Hunchers, and the Crossers. *Slinkers* shove their hips forward in the chair and round their lower backs, actually sitting on their spines. *Hunchers* (often computer users) round their shoulders and push the chin forward, creating

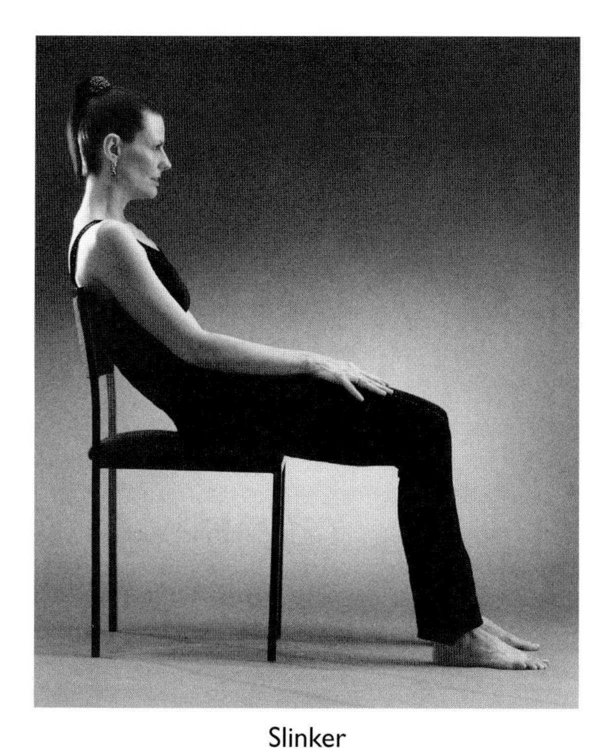
Slinker

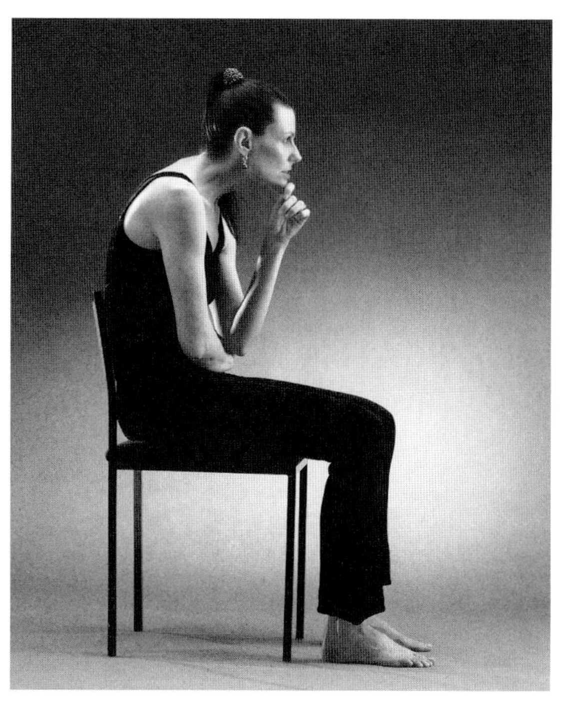
Huncher

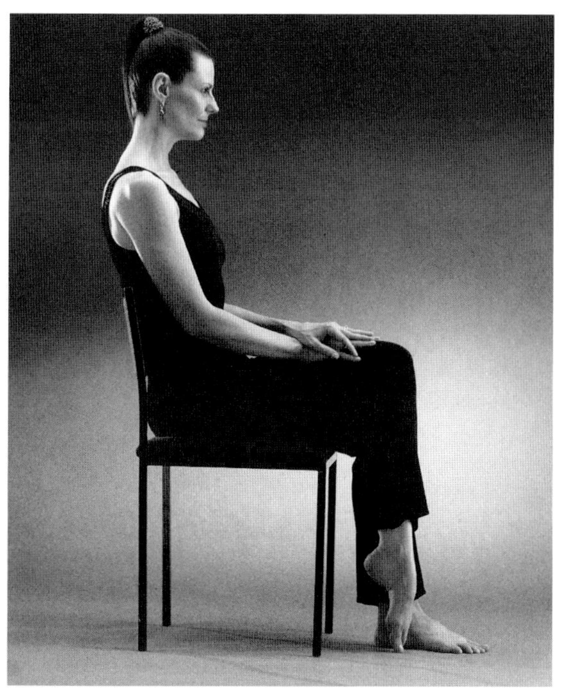
Crosser

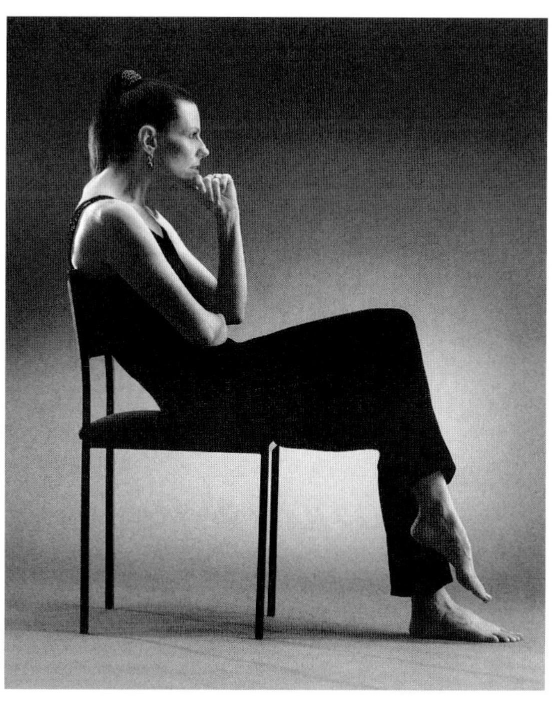
Combined Slinker/Huncher/Crosser

neck and shoulder tension. *Crossers* cross their thighs, throwing the spine a curve. Some of us are a combination of two or even all three syndromes. Which do you tend toward?

Before we learn how to sit well, let's discover how *not* to sit. First, sit on your hands and find the sitting bones (the big bones cushioned by the buttocks). Let's see what happens when we turn the pelvis under and roll backward off these bones: They disappear, and we become instant Slinkers. Once we lose contact with the sit-bones, we are sitting on the spine and stressing the discs.

Now let's feel what happens to Crossers. Still sitting on your hands, cross your thighs. What happens? Are you favoring one sit-bone over the other? Which one? What does this do to the spine? Can you feel how the single action of crossing the thighs also simultaneously dumps the weight into the sit-bone of the bottom leg, skews the spine, and reduces circulation?

Now let's live briefly as a Huncher. Round the shoulders and stick your neck out. Where do you feel this? Probably in that stress repository so many of us share—the back of the neck and shoulders. Spending a few minutes in any of these positions may seem harmless, but consider the cumulative toll of returning to the same contortion hour after unconscious hour, day after day, decade after decade, over a lifetime. No wonder we hurt. No wonder we're tired.

Active Sitting

Sitting well is simpler than the convolutions we've devised through the years, but like any habit, it requires practice. First, uncross your legs. Sit *on top* of your sitting bones, never *behind* them. In time you won't need your hands to find these bones. Like the metal contacts on the base of a cell phone that recharges in its cradle, your sitting bones will connect with the seat to charge up your body.

Once you have your base, the rest is simple. Line up your ears with the shoulders, and the shoulders with (not in front of, and not in back of) the hips. In short: head over heart over hips. Finally, simply push the top of your head away from your seat.

One student uses active sitting during a task she had never enjoyed:

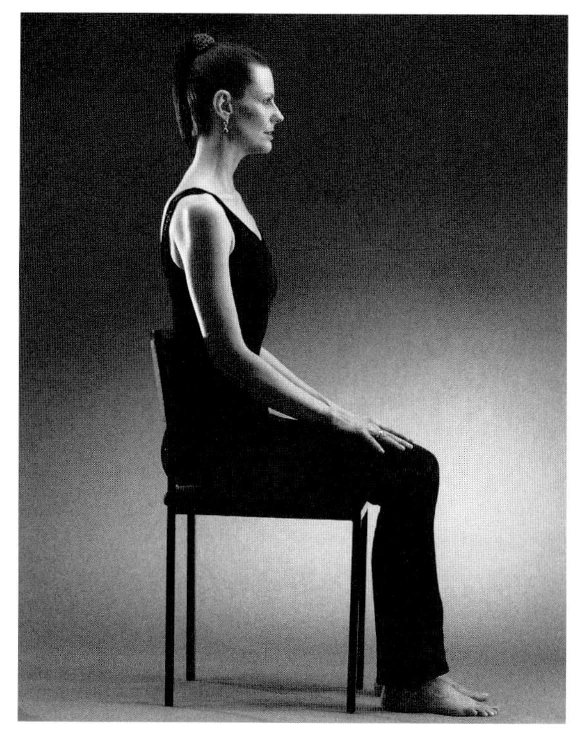
Active Sitting

paying bills. Now, the longer she sits and the more bills she pays, the more energy she discovers. It makes perfect, palpable sense. In active sitting, we're using muscles to support bones, thus sending more blood and oxygen around the body and burning more fuel. Plus, we're giving our organs the room they need to function efficiently. How can we expect the organs to do their jobs well if we're compressing them all the time?

Active sitting isn't just good posture, it's Yoganetics. *It is an activity, a process of extension, not a position we assume and hold.* As with yoga, the results of practice are both immediate and cumulative. While you sit there doubling the calories you burn, you probably feel better already, but the long-term effects build on this as the body gets stronger and more open.

Active sitting is its own reward.

Anatomy of a Reflex

When you are learning a new skill such as active sitting, constant monitoring and effort may be needed. Changing behavior is a three-step process in which you:

1. Become aware of your tendencies
2. Catch yourself in the act
3. Replace old habits with smart ones

Again, any reminders that you can create, from rubber bands to Post-it notes, will cue you to remember what you are doing.

Where else might we use this potent technique? One woman practices in the bleachers at her grandson's basketball games. "It really keeps the back from getting all 'bent out of shape,'" she notes, since bleachers offer no support for the spine. "This really is the way to go!"

Being in an audience is a wonderful cue to practice—whether at a concert, the theater, a sporting event, church, or temple. Any meeting will do, and you may find yourself listening and participating on a new level. Sitting down to a meal is another natural and regular cue. Your digestive tract will thank you.

Let this be your sign to recharge: whenever sitting bones meet seat. With practice, active sitting will become reflexive, and your body itself will be the reminder. When I get off-kilter, an inner alarm in the form of discomfort goes off. I have learned to pay attention. If I ignore it, the alarm just gets louder until I adjust.

Like any new form of exercise, sitting actively may tire you at first. After all, rather than hanging on your bones, you are asking core muscles you haven't been using to start supporting you. The more you use these muscles, the stronger they become, and the more you can rely on them. Once the technique becomes a reflex, it will feel effortless and energizing.

Dream Chair

No matter how active a sitter you are, proper alignment is impossible to maintain in the kind of cushy chairs that clutter living rooms across the land. Our sofas and easy chairs behave more like quicksand than support—sucking us down rather than bolstering us up.

Befriend a straight chair. Meanwhile, consider replacing furniture that is not body-friendly. Ergonomic choices don't have to be pricey, and the return is priceless, especially if you work at a desk or spend a large part of your day seated. Everyone should have at least one chair to call "home." That means it feels heavenly to be there and gives you the support your body craves.

Just like a coat, the chair needs to fit your body and should be adjustable if you're going to share it with others. Look for firmness beneath the hips and lumbar support behind the waist, as well as proper arm height, seat height, and depth (length of leg).

The investment you make will return to you in the form of well-being. There's no going back once you experience furniture that serves rather than saps you.

Dynamic Duo

Like peanut butter and jelly, Fred and Ginger, popcorn and movies, two techniques you are learning make an exquisite pair.

Experiment: Set aside five minutes at your desk to combine active sitting with path breathing. How do they affect one another?

"One paves the way for the other," says a student who found that active sitting makes path breathing possible and vice versa. Because we have made room in the body through active sitting, we can travel the path. Because we are traveling the path, the spine is supported. A perfect symbiosis.

"Path breathing while active sitting feels more expansive than lying down," says another practitioner. Without a floor against the spine, the experience becomes fully three-dimensional as "the torso feels more opened—outward to the sides as well as front to back."

"It seems like a very effective, quick meditation," says another. This duo has a powerhouse effect, however tired or upset you may feel. Just plug in through your sit-bones, line yourself up, push the crown from your core, and let the breath rain down through you to rise again from the depths of your being.

Active sitting and path breathing will support you when you need it the most. They are yours within, just a choice away, and will return you to a place of strength. Let their fusion imbue your life with power and grace.

Nine

Growing Up

She saw no one in the cave. But the moment she stood upright she had a marvellous sense that she was in the secret of the earth and all its ways.

George MacDonald, *The Golden Key*

We may be world travelers with multiple degrees, but in terms of how well we know the body that takes us everywhere, we're babies. Take a look around and see what all the grown-ups are doing. Watch shoppers in line at the grocery store. Become a spy at cocktail parties and restaurants and meetings—wherever people are standing. We skew our spines into question marks, favor one leg over another, then wonder why we feel ill at ease.

First, we're not giving our organs the space they need to work efficiently. Second, we're twisting ourselves into contortions that cut off the flow within. Assiduously taught us by the popular media, these postures may look wonderfully interesting and asymmetrical through the camera lens, but they are destructive. Finally, we're not getting enough exercise—or exercise of the right kind.

Eternal beginners all, it's never too late to re-educate the body. As babies, we made the great shift from crawling on all fours to walking upright. Considering the epidemic of joint and back pain among us, we have yet to master the two-footed realm. Let's continue our evolution as bipeds and discover a way of standing and walking that empowers rather than depletes us.

In short, let's grow up.

The Shift to Vertical

Now comes the translation of all we are learning from the horizontal to the vertical. The alignment the earth has been teaching us each time we lie down to practice can transfer to our standing lives, but only if we monitor the behavior we've been ignoring.

Experiment: Measure your height first thing in the morning and last thing at night. When are you taller? By how much?

"Can this be right?" says one student. "Isaac Newton, say it isn't so!"

You may be surprised to learn that you are taller in the morning. It's common to lose between a half-inch and an inch in height over the course of a single day. Why? Two reasons: (1) gravity, and (2) our response to gravity.

We can't do anything about gravity, but we can manage our response to it. During the day, the weight of the head, arms, shoulders, and upper body presses down on the spine's natural curves. The spine gets curvier, and the discs, the little pillows between vertebrae, get compressed. At night when we're horizontal, the spine elongates and our discs fill up again with fluid. So in the morning—magic!—we rise from our beds taller than when we lay down.

If height loss occurs in the microcosm of one day, consider what happens over a lifetime of days, decade after decade.

A quick anatomy lesson. The spine is a snake with three main curves: cervical (neck), thoracic (ribs), and lumbar (lower back). These curves form an elongated "S" shape. The longer we walk around on Earth, the deeper our "S" curves tend to become—and the deeper our curves, the shorter we get. It is normal (but not natural) to lose height as we age. Now for another surprise.

Experiment: Enlist a friend to measure the length of your spine twice. First, stand tall and measure from the base of the skull (the indentation where skull meets neck) to the bottom of the coccyx (tailbone). Then bend your knees, walk your hands down your legs, and hang forward. Measure again, base of skull to bottom of coccyx. In which position is the spine longer? By how much?

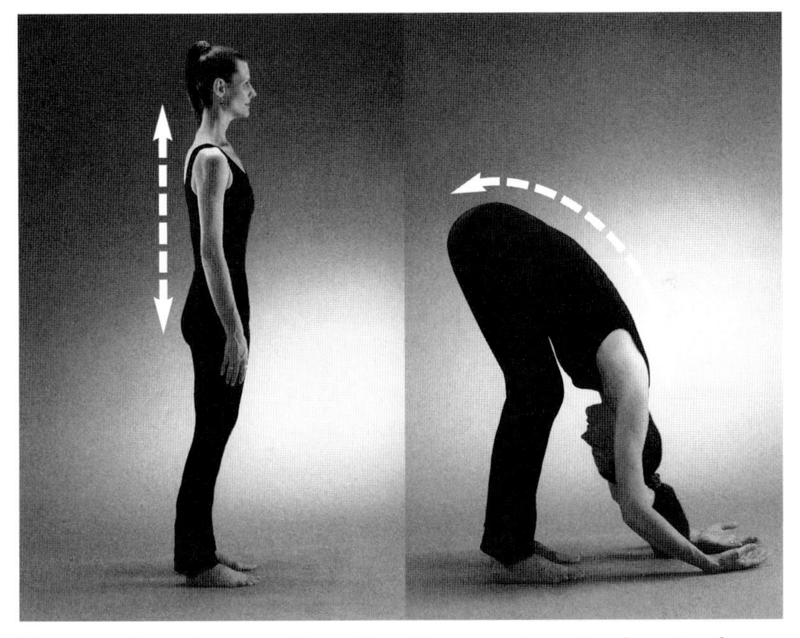

Measure the spine standing tall. Measure the spine hanging forward.

Generally, the spine is between four and seven inches longer when bent over. Why? When we fold forward from the hips, our vertebrae rise to the surface and we discover the spine's true length. In contrast, when we're standing, we've got our curves on, so the spine measures shorter.

That differential—between the spine's actual length and its length when we're "wearing" our curves—we call the available growing space (AGS). That number is our play space, ours to reclaim, millimeter by millimeter. It's not unusual for people to become taller as they learn to elongate their compressed curves and unfurl to their natural height. Many notice they have to reset their rearview mirror after a single session of Yoganetics. In time some regain the height they have lost since they were teenagers. Some set new records. Just ask the sixty-eight-year-old grandmother who gained one and a half inches to top five feet for the first time in her life! Or my seven-foot husband, who has begun bumping his head on doorways again.

Now, we wouldn't want to reclaim our AGS completely. We need our curves, because they serve as shock absorbers that help prevent injury. Our goal is to lengthen rather than eliminate them. To do this, we focus on the secondary curves, behind the neck (cervical) and behind the waist (lumbar), where we tend to lose our height. They are called "secondary" because we weren't born with them. These curves developed when we were toddlers in response to the shift from crawling to standing and walking.

Bottom-up Standing

To learn how to stand again, let's start with the foundation. Our feet take us everywhere, yet they feel like strangers. Maybe it's because they're farthest from our brain. But consider this: They have been there for us every step of the way, quietly bearing us along the pathway of our life. It's time we befriended them.

Experiment: Spy on yourself next time you're waiting in line. Are you standing mainly on one foot? Now look around you at the other standing people. Are they favoring one leg?

It's amazing how we bipeds aren't using the feet we have risen to. Many of us rely on just half of ourselves much of the time. When we favor one leg, what happens to the spine? Stand up and see. It skews laterally, a temporary sort of scoliosis. And it's often the same side we favor, neglecting the other.

We'll take a three-step approach to re-educating the feet. The first lesson is to use both of them. Love them equally and make it illegal to stand on one. Second, notice where your inside anklebones are. Are they falling inward toward each other, depressing the arches? Does your weight tend toward the big toe? Start by pulling your ankles back over your feet. This will lift the arches up and distribute your weight more evenly. Spread and lengthen the toes, your personal root system, paying special attention to the little guys—the much neglected fourth and fifth toes.

Third, imagine you're on the beach leaving a footprint in warm sand. Is your weight falling more into the front or back of the foot? If you're like most people, you'd leave a deeper imprint with your heels than with your toes. Try a triangular approach, your weight falling equally into the (1) big toe, (2) little toe, and (3) heel. Triangulation provides a stronger, more dynamic platform to support the body.

Now walk slowly around the room. Are you back to your old habits? Consider the thousands of steps you take each day. Or if you run or do aerobics, consider this: Four times your weight is pounding on your joints eighty times a minute. If your alignment is wrong, your whole body suffers. Knee and back trouble often have roots in the feet.

To strengthen your feet, go barefoot, triangulating as you pad around your home. Every day slip off your shoes and integrate the two following exercises into your life.

Towel Grab

Keep a hand towel handy and do this every time you go to the bathroom. Place the towel on the floor just in front of your toes. Now, grabbing with all ten toes, scrunch the towel until it's under your feet. Then reverse, using a pushing motion until the towel is in front of the feet again.

Sky Writing

Take a break from work and do something productive! Elevate your feet on your desk, or better yet, lie down and bend your knees over your chest. Now write the alphabet in the air, thinking of each toe as a separate paintbrush. Once you feel fluent, write a message to someone across the room and see if you're legible yet.

A brief note on shoes, those oft-strange cages we strap to the ends of our legs. If you invest in your feet, your entire body will thank you. Look for comfort and support, and shop late in the afternoon, when feet are most likely to swell. Many of us have been buying shoes for the eyes. Next time, buy for your feet—as if you are grateful to them for bringing you this far. They will respond in kind.

What Is Your Leading Center?

Now that you are two-footed, the next step is to discover your leading center.

Experiment: Stand profile in front of a mirror and close your eyes. Imagine you are exhausted, and let your body fall into the position it favors when fatigued. Now open your eyes and, without turning your head, glance sideways in the mirror. See through to your bones, as if you were an X-ray machine. What part of you would cross a finish line first? Is it your head, heart, or hips?

When we stand, we may think we're vertical, but most of us are a wildly idiosyncratic zig-zag under construction since infancy.

Head Leaders are often desk workers, especially men. In any zig-zag, something goes forward (in this case, the head), and something goes back to counterbalance it (the chest). By leading with the head, people automatically counterbalance by holding back in the heart. This posture accentuates the cervical curve, creating neck and shoulder tension. Stick your neck out and see for yourself.

Heart Leaders lead with their chests—but again, if something goes forward (the heart), something goes back to counterbalance (the hips). This is the "dumb blonde" stance perfected by Hollywood and delivered to our living rooms nightly. It is the famous "T&A" carriage from Broadway's *Chorus Line*. And it leads directly to middle-back pain.

Hip Leaders resemble fashion models who are trained to lead with the pelvis. But in the body's zig-zag wisdom, if something goes forward (the hips), something will go back to counterbalance it (the heart). When the lower body leads, the upper body falls back. This stance deepens the lumbar curve and generates low-back problems.

As you stand and walk around, experiment by exaggerating any one of these three postures, and you will discover on a visceral level what part of the spine this behavior will harm over time, and what curve it will deepen. (Here we arrive at the paradox of high heels: In the short term they make you taller, but ultimately they shorten you by increasing your zig-zag.)

Your sitting posture may well carry over to your standing behavior. If in chapter 8 you discovered that you are a Huncher—jutting the chin

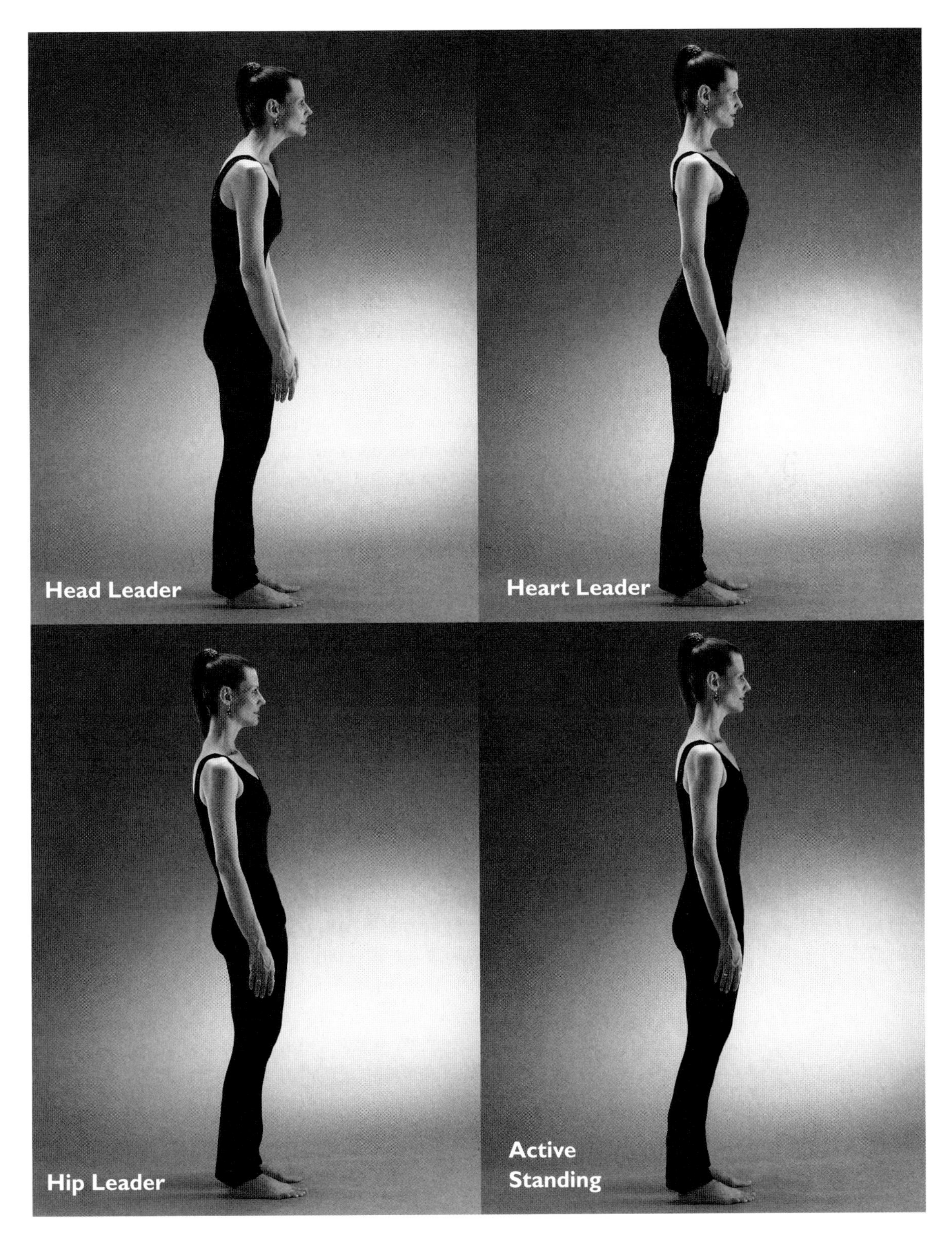
Head Leader
Heart Leader
Hip Leader
Active
Standing

forward and rounding the shoulders—it's no surprise that when you rise from your chair, you are a Head Leader. If you're a Slinker and push the hips forward in your seat, you are probably a walking Hip Leader as well.

These are, of course, very general categories, but most people fall into one of them. Some of us combine two centers, but one will predominate, as with the Hip Leader whose head is a secondary leading center.

Active Standing

Once you know your tendencies, you are in a position to change them. In active standing, you use muscles to support your body, instead of leaning on counters and pillars and your own dear bones. Just follow this three-step process.

Experiment:

1. Stand profile in front of a mirror, triangulating on two feet with soft knees.
2. Line up your head over your heart center over your hips, like a triple ice cream cone or a triad chord.
3. Push the crown of your head out of your belly and into the sky. Point the tips of your ears upward (like Spock on *Star Trek*).

Some people refer to this alignment as ears in line with shoulders in line with hips. Others prefer the concept of head over heart over hips. Some people are helped by visualizing themselves hanging from their hair. For me, active standing is a birthing process, giving birth to undiscovered height from deep in the core of the body. I simply center myself in the cave, then push my crown skyward. The rest falls into place.

The payoff is immediate. "I was standing in line at the store," says one practitioner. "One foot was resting on the bottom shelf of the shopping cart, and my upper body was draped over the handles. My lower back was hurting. I stood on both feet, aligned my body, and practiced 'active standing' for the next five minutes until my turn came up in line. It felt a bit rigid at first. However, I then noticed the pain in my lower back was easing. I felt more alert—no longer a wet noodle draped over the shopping cart. I only wish I had the experience on videotape!"

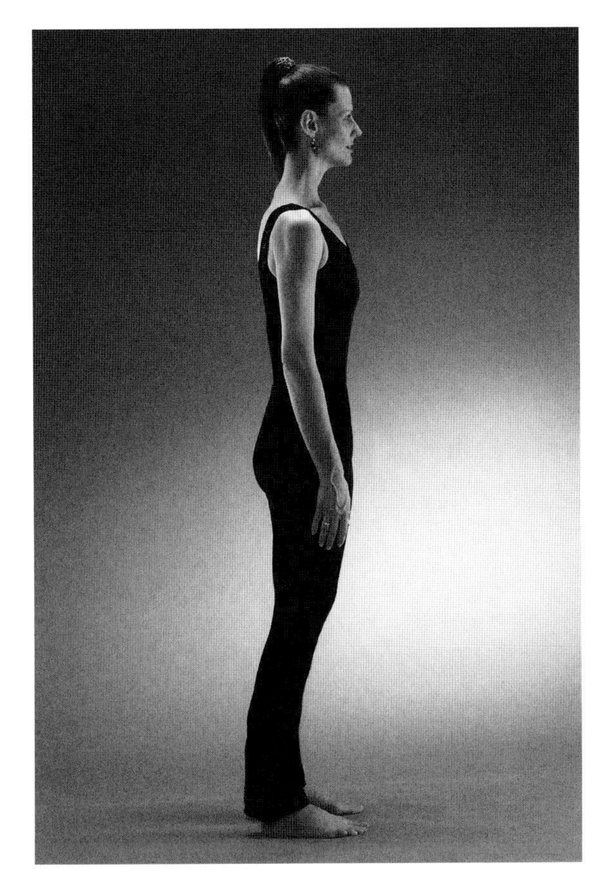

Active Standing:
Head over heart over hips

Another student did active standing in the drugstore. "I felt more room in my torso, my lungs filled more fully, and I was more aware of giving my body the right space to live in. I felt more energetic and precise." Another practiced while having a conversation "for an extended period. What a difference—not nearly so tiring. It's actually relaxing!"

Active standing gives energy while using energy. Just like active sitting, standing properly is a natural metabolism raiser because it burns twice the calories as hanging on the bones. Don't get discouraged if at first it feels unnatural. "I practiced this over and over these past few days," says one young woman. "What a difference! At first it felt awkward. But very quickly it begins to feel comfortable. Now that I am standing in a balanced form, there is no one place that squeaks out pain."

Until you have replaced the former reflex with the smarter one, you'll notice yourself lapsing into the old and recreating the new again and again. That's a sign you're on track, transforming yourself moment by moment into a new way of being.

Spy Games

It's always interesting to notice the choices that people are making. Lessons are everywhere around us. Out of the thousands we surveyed, my students found that *97 percent of us are standing improperly.*

Experiment: **Next time you're out and about, conduct a random survey of standing people. First, fold a page into four sections, then put a heading on each: One-Footers, Head Leaders, Heart Leaders, Hip Leaders. Use the back of your sheet for Active Standers (if you find any). Make a mark in each section until you have a hundred samples, then tally your percentages.**

"Sloppy, sloppy, sloppy!" says one spy. "I can't believe how many people have bad standing and sitting postures. And it feels so bad to sit and stand so bad!"

"Almost all the people I observed were standing with weight shifted to one leg," says another. "I did see two people with both feet planted evenly, but they had their shoulders back and pelvis forward."

Holidays are great times to spy on your family at large. "One was at the sink doing dishes, leaning more on one leg than the other, while one was drying dishes leaning her back against the counter to hold herself up," says another. "In the family room, people were all slouched into chairs and the sofa watching football games."

Sound familiar? And exhausting. So often, the very people who make poor physical choices are also tired and grumpy. If only they knew that sitting and standing differently could make a difference in how they feel *inside.*

Our job is not to criticize or "fix" others but just to notice them, be inspired by them, and apply our learning to ourselves. Like emotions, posture is contagious. If we do our work, those around us are affected, and they frequently respond by realigning themselves.

We can transform the body one decision at a time—from a thing to lug around to an energy field that recharges us. The choice is ours right now. As I sit here writing and you sit here reading, we can choose to empower ourselves. And when we get up from our chairs and move on to what's next, we choose again and again. A new life unfurls within us wherever we go.

Ten

Integration

It was the best place to be, thought Wilbur, this warm delicious cellar, with the garrulous geese, the changing seasons, the heat of the sun, the passage of swallows, the nearness of rats, the sameness of sheep, the love of spiders, the smell of manure, and the glory of everything.

E. B. WHITE, *CHARLOTTE'S WEB*

Our mission is nothing short of integration, as we embody on a visceral level all that we are discovering physically, intellectually, emotionally, and spiritually. Our purpose is to unite feeling and form, breath and motion, the divine and the divorced parts of ourselves, until mind, body, and spirit are one in every moment of life.

This sense of integration is honed as we deepen our experience of the body's core. No longer flailing in space far from the brain, the limbs become anchored in the center, like a starfish. And the body starts operating from the core outward in everything it does.

Experiment: Next sunny day, find a bench and watch people move. Whether you're spying on runners or dog-walkers, don't be distracted by the outer motion. Look for the source of the motion, the place in the body where the movement begins.

Where is the hub of all the hubbub? Notice how high up people center themselves. We tend to be front-and-upper-body oriented, centering ourselves in the chest or head. Teetering way above our feet, we lack a firm connection not only to our primal core, but to the earth beneath. It's a wonder we don't fall over.

The Middle of the Story

Middles aren't easy places. What comes to mind when we think of middle children, middle age, midlife crisis? For choreographers, writers, artists, or any of us who have ever started to create something with energy that fizzled mid-task, the real work lies in the middle of the project. Beginnings are exciting, endings often inspired, but betwixt and between is the body of the story we're telling.

Bodywise, the middle is an especially ambiguous place. It's the least bony, the most fluid, and structurally the weakest part of us. While our arms may have hefted suitcases to all corners of the earth, and our legs tramped every step, the core is missing. Some of us compensate by "chesting" it, with great bravado pulling up and away from our center, tensing our shoulders, and even bouncing when we walk. Others of us collapse—the spine slumping into a question mark that casts our gaze down, down, down.

There is a middle ground. Why is finding it so important, and so difficult? Consider the geography of the bones. If the big bony continent of the rib cage is North America, and the big bony continent of the pelvis is South America, all that connects these land masses is the Central American isthmus of the lumbar spine. That sliver of lumbar land is subject to the ever-changing stormy seas of our middle body. Is it any wonder the lower back is stressed?

To extend the metaphor, if the waist is a kind of equator below which another language is spoken, maybe we should spend some time down there and become fluent. Because, as foreign as this place may feel at first, in the midst of us is an oasis. Lure yourself here throughout the day as you sit, stand, and breathe. Then watch what happens. In time you'll move south because the climate is so amazing.

Cultivating Hara

Translated from the Japanese, *Hara* means "belly." We're not talking about the organ of the stomach, but about the actual center of the body, its specific midpoint. It lies halfway between head and toes, halfway between the left and right sides, and halfway between the front and back of the body. We have found this place again and again in our yoga practice, but we need to return here in everything we do.

In *Charlotte's Web,* Wilbur makes his home in the cellar, euphorically described by E. B. White at the beginning of this chapter. In Yoganetics we call it the cave. It is a safe and sacred place that provides shelter from storms and a sanctuary in which to nurture ourselves, to discover our own glistening depths, and to dream of what's beyond. "Here, everything concerned with the Greater Life is conceived, carried and born," wrote philosopher and psychotherapist Karlfried Graf Von Dürckheim in *Hara: The Vital Centre of Man.* "Here all renewal has its beginning and from here alone it ascends."

In the following exercise, we will re-establish the gravitational center and begin the process of cultivating Hara. Notice how much lower this place is than where we usually venture. It's in the deep end of the swimming pool. In women it's where the womb is, or was. It's where we grew in our own mother's body. It's the center of the star we are.

Finding the Star

Lie down on your back with knees bent or straight, and close your eyes. Let the spine lengthen, especially the curves behind the neck and waist. Place your hands on top of the belly between your hipbones. With one hand find the navel, and with the other the top of the pubic bone. Now locate the midpoint between these two places. Press one hand gently downward here, and drop your attention at this level just in front of your spine, below the surface abdominal muscles. This is your gravitational center, in the core of the body. Imagine your five points (legs, arms, spine) connected to this place, like a star.

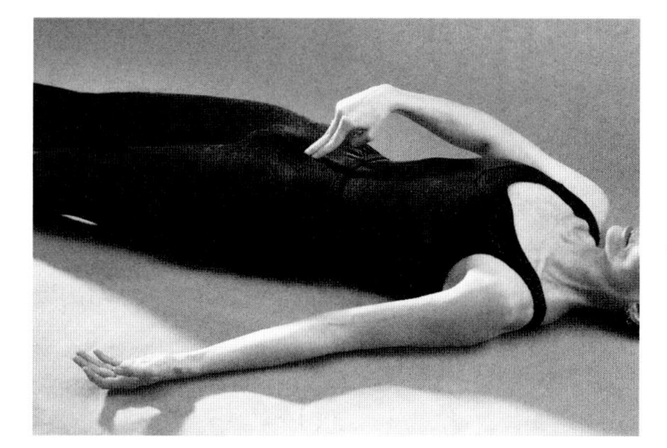

The center of the star

Move into your Hara and make it your own, as if you could see and hear from this depth. Close your eyes and imagine that your favorite chair awaits you in the center of your body. Sit down. Put your feet up. Unpack your bags. And begin to live from here.

Keep reading through the next two paragraphs as you physically follow the suggestions. Sitting up on your sit-bones, push the top of your head out of your belly and into the sky. Staying connected, press through your legs and feet down into the earth and rise from your chair. Still centered, with your whole consciousness rooted deep in your core, walk across the room.

As you walk, feel how the strong stem of your spine extends from the core of the trunk upward through the crown. Then imagine growing roots down your thighs from inside your belly, and feel the earth through the soles of your feet. Every step you take, feel the earth from deep inside your core. This connection will nourish you. Just as trees take water from the soil through their trunks and into their branches, we re-energize ourselves from the bottom up. Through our legs, we are connected from our belly to the belly of the earth, so that we become, as the Bible says, like trees walking.

How does that feel? How does your spine feel, specifically your lower back? Do you feel taller, yet more grounded? Life would be different if we returned our sense of center to its actual depth. Imagine running, lifting, climbing stairs with Hara, instead of flinging ourselves at the world from a height above the collar.

Experiment: While doing any household chore—sweeping, straightening, lifting, dishwashing—push your head out of your belly and source the movement from the cave. From this depth of center, all life (and limb and motion) is connected. How does practicing Hara affect you and your task?

People notice many benefits, among them less back pain. "Any lifting of heavy boxes, laundry, etc., was much easier working from the 'cave' and took stress and strain off my lower back," says one student. Another practiced while vacuuming and "found that by sourcing the movement from the belly, my back and shoulders did not get as tired."

"As I straightened the house," says another, "I was less tired, had more stamina, and no back pain." Practicing Hara is naturally strengthening and restorative because we rely more on the abdominals and less on the back. This may sound obvious, but as the belly gets stronger, the back undergoes less wear and tear.

As our sense of Hara grows, this core connection stabilizes the whole body. One woman practiced while painting her kitchen. "My balance going up and down the ladder improved. Wow! You *can* teach an old dog new tricks!" Another used it to clean her deck. "I felt a greater sense of balance and stability. Also, I noticed that the work seemed easier."

The work does get easier because the body gets better coordinated. "I feel taller and more elegant in my movements," says one student. Another notices that she feels not only more graceful but more unified, "as if my legs were attached to my navel!" Another is amazed to find that her body "feels more connected with all its parts." Coordination is the beginning of grace, made possible through integration.

With Hara, the arms and legs plug into a greater power source, and we begin to discover how strong we really are. The experience transcends the merely muscular.

"The strength experienced is the strength of an inner firmness not created by us, but given to us," says Von Dürckheim. "Even more important than this new outward strength is the experience of the mysterious power itself. It is not a power one *has,* but a power in which one *stands.*"

We begin developing Hara by active sitting and standing from the center outward. In time the experience goes beyond the postural to re-create us from within. We not only stand differently, notes Von Dürckheim, but we stand as a different person, for with Hara we are not who we were when we yanked ourselves upward or sagged weakly downward.

In Japan it is said that a person either has Hara or does not. But Hara can be developed—at first imaginatively, then viscerally—by finding the gravitational center, linking the limbs to it, then sourcing every position and motion from this powerful place. As you practice Yoganetics, work from this depth, from the core outward. Walk from here and talk from here. Live (and sing and vacuum) from your Hara, where your star shines out in all directions.

The Left-and-Rightness of Things

Hara is integrative in a very deep and primal way. But there is also some finer motor work to do to reintegrate the two sides of the body. From scissors to stick shifts, we live in a world that is geared to the right. Maybe you haven't noticed the way doors are hung and drinking fountains are positioned to favor right-handers. But the lefties among us (who in the early twentieth century were schooled to switch and write right) are certainly aware of the "rightness" of things.

Our language reflects the bias. We're not wrong, but right, and it is our rightful duty and birthright to be right-minded and demand our rights. The lefties are, well, left. Left behind. Left over. Plagued with two left feet. Consider the adage, "The right hand doesn't know what the left is doing." It describes organizations that aren't well coordinated. But it also applies to the way our body has become divided. One side feels familiar, the other is a stranger we've seen lurking about but never befriended.

In competitive sports we cultivate lopsidedness—using a baseball bat, tennis racket, golf club, or hockey stick to move a ball around. Our whole physical education system is based on learning games that promote fun and teamwork, but imbalance the body. Noncompetitive activities that foster integration, such as dance and yoga, tend to be overlooked.

It's never too late, however, to begin to marry the two sides of our body. We start small, with a formal introduction. The hand you write with is your "dominant" hand. The other hand is your "helper" hand. Your first assignment is to let the "helper" actually help!

Experiment: **Next time the phone rings, pick it up with your helper. Use your helper to open the door, clean off your desk, vacuum, and sweep. Notice how unfamiliar or weak this side feels? You may also find that your task becomes a whole new activity.**

Reassign unimportant tasks—tossing stuff in the wastebasket, switching on lights—to your neglected side. (It helps not to be in a hurry.) In time graduate to finer motor skills. Use your helper to dial the phone, count change, and write the grocery list.

One day when you're alone, try eating with the other hand. It's a little like learning manners all over, but using your helper will slow down the dining experience—and facilitate better digestion. The slower you eat, the more in touch you will be with how full you feel, reducing your intake of food and fostering natural weight loss.

If you use a computer, place your mouse on the other side. I just switched mine over and feel suddenly like a child learning a new skill. The whole task of writing and editing is new. I may not be rolling down the page as fast as usual, but I'm certainly more aware of my journey.

A lot of life we can simply delegate to the other side. By letting our helper help, we stimulate neural pathways, strengthening and quickening them. So not only does our body get better coordinated, but our reflexes get faster. And we travel the road to wholeness.

Recovering from Illness and Injury

Integration is also a process of making peace with the past so that we can move fully into the present. Bodywise, that means welcoming places of trauma, illness, or injury back into our consciousness. If you've ever been injured (and who hasn't?) you may still have unfinished business at the site of the injury. Scar tissue may not be the only thing you left behind. It's likely that you abandoned the place that hurt, like a room you moved out of because the view was bad.

When we hurt, our tendency is to withdraw our attention from the place of pain. That's a natural response, but a short-term solution. In the long run, abandoning the site of an injury will retard the healing process, and it may be years, decades, or even a lifetime before we realize that we've lost part of ourselves in the process.

I've been through this in my own body. And I see it over and over in my classes—people who can't breathe below a particular place, or whose musculature is locked, or who can't access certain parts. Underneath these symptoms is usually a story. Whether it's a car wreck, surgery, or a simple fall, trauma is trauma. The body remembers, *especially* if the conscious mind has forgotten.

While Yoganetics is not a substitute for counseling or medical attention, it can play a role in the therapeutic process. If there is a place in you that feels vague or uncomfortable or still painful, it's never too late to revisit and reclaim it. Like the runt of the litter who's been ignored, this part of your body has been starved for attention. Welcome it back to the fold.

Reintegration is a process, so be patient. The first step is simply to bring your awareness back to the site you abandoned. Healing begins the moment we revisit this place, bridging the separation within us and beginning the round-trip journey home.

Just as in the treasure tension hunt (see the Inner Voyage, chapter 3), we will move through the body here, following our sensations into any discomfort we discover. Then we'll invite the wind along the path. Starting from the heart center, simply direct the pathway to the part of your body that needs attention. By breathing directly into the precise size and shape of your discomfort, you will feel it respond, begin to shift, and eventually dissolve. Record the following paragraph, or read it quietly, pausing between sentences to close your eyes and feel the way. Take at least five minutes for this journey every day, or as often as you like.

The Round Trip

Lie down or sit comfortably, close your eyes, and relax. Surrender the weight of the body, and let your mind follow your sensations, like a child following clues on a treasure hunt. As if there were an opening at the crown of the head, let light pour through it behind the face. Relax the features.

Follow the light through the open throat and into the body. Let it move through every part of you, shining away darkness as you roam the body from head through toenails. Linger anywhere you feel discomfort, an old injury, or no sensation at all. Just linger. There's nothing to do.

Feel the exact size of this place. Feel its shape. Does it have a color? Now just rest here, entirely safe, noticing whether the shape is shifting in any way. Starting from the heart center, inhale and direct the path of breath into this place. Feel it filling with wind and light. Exhale and watch it deflate a little as the breath leads the way and you begin the process of release.

Keep breathing and watching and feeling your way along. Eventually, like the rock worn away by the river, discomfort will dissolve in the flowing current of your breath and the healing light of your attention.

What you discover may surprise you. "The other night I woke up because my hip joint and foot were hurting very badly," says one woman. "I could not fall asleep again. Then I started my deep breathing and within three to four breaths, a pleasant warmth spread through the joint and the pain was gone. I did the same with the arch of my foot—same result! I was so excited about it, and in the morning I could hardly believe it. This feeling has now spread to my overall well-being."

Our bodies have much to teach us if we are present enough to listen. Come back to the place you abandoned and be whole.

Connecting the Dots

We are in a process of connecting the dots. By following one dot to the next and the next, we discover the bigger picture. Keep looking for new connections inside, each one a breakthrough: the relationship between the brow and the lower back, the alliance between the arches and the inner thighs. You'll find your own remarkable links, and in time the once-separated dots will become a far-flung constellation in the great space you are becoming.

As connections are made, distinctions disappear. The line between form and content begins to blur. Just as the belly falls into the spine on the exhalation, eventually the front and back become so intimate that the separation between them gives way. The belly becomes the spine, and they are one. What support there is in this union!

As we exhale, not only does the front fall into the back, but the lower moves into the upper. The inner body knows no such division as "upper" and "lower." Only the outer body, subject to whims of fashion designers, is divided—sequestered and lashed at the waist with elastic bands and belts of all sorts. We must learn to surrender these separations with every breath we take.

I once asked my yoga teacher, Eric Beeler, what his goal in the work was. "To disappear," he calmly replied. This perplexed me, since at the time I was an adolescent trying to emerge from my cocoon. Over the years in my own practice, I have begun to understand what he meant.

"Leave no trace," says the mystic. The poet vanishes into the poem the way stitches disappear into a piece of clothing. The yogi vanishes into the pose in the same way. The deeper the experience, the more transparent the body. The front becomes the back, the lower becomes the upper, and we disappear. We are no longer *doing* yoga. We *are* yoga—one with the breath, the pose, and the spirit that infuses it.

We're marrying the abandoned to the acknowledged, the left to the right, the upper to the lower, the front to the back, all body parts to the center, and that center to the earth from which we are made. Maybe it's time to give up the fight to remain divided, to recognize that we are one, not only with our body but with others, as we cross the bridge to one another.

When we hear music, our heartbeat and respiration respond to its tempo, slowing down or speeding up in kind. When we become intimate with another person, our hearts join in rhythm, as does our breath. These connections are natural and sympathetic responses, much like women living in the same house whose periods begin to coincide.

In a yoga class, the whole room can become one heartbeat, one breath drawn and released through the bigger wind tunnel that we are. After all, the boundary of our skin does not really separate us from one another. Skin is porous, more window screen than wall, through which the wind can pass. At first we reduced our wind tunnel to the size of a straw to narrow and lengthen the breath. Then we enlarged it to the shape of our torso, between the power center and the heart center. Once Hara has become firmly established, we can close our eyes and move through the porous border of the body into the space beyond, expanding the wind tunnel as far as we dare. As we inhale, we can fill a room, fill a circus tent, fill a sky.

When I am teaching, I sometimes imagine the roomful of us rooted together through our centers like a great redwood forest. The sound of the wind is thrilling as it roams through every leaf on every tree. But the secret of the forest lies not in its shimmering leaves and bending branches, however dazzling. The secret lies just out of sight, below the earth. Each tree stands, not because of its own root system, but because of a complex intertwining of roots with surrounding trees. It is this invisible connection that renders the forest its height and every tree its seemingly singular life.

We are all connected. As in the forest, our connection exists out of sight. The fox in *The Little Prince* puts it perfectly: "What is essential is invisible to the eye." Or as my yoga teacher suggested, our job is to disappear.

That's where we're heading, from the visible to the invisible, and it's one reason we do the work with the eyes closed. The body is nothing more than a vibrating field of energy. As we become attuned to this energy, our borders blur and we become transparent, moving through imagined boundaries to encompass the space on the other side of the skin. The distinction between inner and outer dissolves. The ticking clock is happening within our expanded awareness, as is the train whistle in the distance, the wind pushing the trees, and the whole swirling sigh of the universe. As our boundaries evaporate, we disappear into something much bigger.

What a paradox: When we vanish, we start to get *really* big. Our education goes not only beyond the mat, but ultimately beyond the body. And so we arrive at another paradox: To move beyond the body, we must first inhabit it fully. As T. S. Eliot said, "In my end is my beginning."

Welcome home.

Health Guide

Yoga Benefits for Specific Conditions

Here is some of what we are learning about a variety of health concerns, culled from a growing body of research and the bodies of Yoganetics students.

AIDS

Yoga can improve the health and quality of life for people with AIDS (PWAs), reports *Yoga Journal.* Studies in Spain, India, Germany, and Africa suggest that yoga can retard the disease while improving mental health and body image. Published studies in the United States show that yoga also addresses the ailments that some PWAs experience, such as substance abuse, depression, anxiety, heart disease, high blood pressure, high cholesterol and blood sugar, headaches, and chronic pain.

Arthritis

Because much of yoga involves non-weight-bearing, breath-based movement, it is easy on the joints and a natural fitness choice for people with arthritis. A recent study at the University of Pennsylvania School of Medicine has shown that yoga significantly increases range of motion while decreasing pain and tenderness in those suffering from osteoarthritis.

One student, a nurse, puts it this way: "By my calculation, [Yoganetics] has saved me twenty dollars in the last eight weeks by decreasing my drug consumption 50 percent. After battling arthritic pain for several years, I have finally found something that makes my muscles feel better than taking medication."

Asthma

Yogic breathing can help reduce asthma attacks. A controlled clinical study at the Northern Colorado Allergy Asthma Clinic suggests that yoga is beneficial for asthma and can reduce use of inhalers.

Yoga increases lung capacity. One woman who suffered a punctured lung convinced her insurance company to cover Yoganetics. "The exercises have increased my peak flow forty liters!" she reports.

Back Pain

Back pain is the single largest cause of employee absenteeism in our country, affecting 80 percent of Americans at some point in their lives. In a nationwide survey of 492 people from every state, researchers found that of all known remedies for common backache—including surgery, manipulation, physical therapy, biofeedback, herbalism, rolfing, and various types of exercise—yoga proved the most effective.

"If a patient were going to do one thing inexpensively, I would tell that patient to go take a yoga course," says orthopedic surgeon Arthur White, a major contributor to the field of spine care.

Yoganetics has demonstrated both short- and long-term benefits. "When I come to class, my back hurts," says one man. "When I leave, it doesn't." As back-healthy habits become established, symptoms may vanish altogether. "I used to have lower-back pain regularly," says a woman in her forties. "That has disappeared."

Cancer

"Yoga can reduce your risk [of breast cancer] by stimulating lymph flow, strengthening the endocrine and immune systems, and improving your attitude toward your body," says *Yoga Journal.*

For those living with cancer, yoga offers assistance in coping with the condition. "Chemotherapy, surgery, and some medications can rob you of mental acuity," says Sue Cohen in *Time* magazine. The fifty-four-year-old accountant and breast-cancer survivor says that "yoga helps compensate for the loss. It impels you to do things you never thought you were capable of doing."

Chronic Pain

According to the American Pain Foundation, more than 50 million Americans suffer from some form of chronic pain. Unlike acute pain, chronic pain may not be associated with an injury. In a study at Texas Tech University that blended yoga and meditation with traditional medical treatment, 79 percent of participants said their condition improved.

Depression

Research indicates that yoga has a beneficial effect on the emotional well-being and mental acuity of those undergoing depression—with no side effects. A Scandinavian study found a 40 percent increase in alpha and theta brain waves, suggesting that yoga helps alleviate depression by increasing "feel-good" endorphins, enkephalins, and serotonin, as well as providing greater access to feelings.

A study at Philadelphia's Jefferson Medical College found that after just one yoga class, levels of cortisol (an indicator of depression when elevated) were significantly reduced.

According to the *New York Times,* "Americans use the yoga mat as a therapist's couch, and often as a church pew." Yoga takes an integrative, inside-out approach to the body that trains more than muscles. Mind, body, and spirit respond to this quality of attention.

Fibromyalgia

Those with fibromyalgia syndrome (FS) respond well to yoga. Research at the Pain Center of the Texas Tech University Health Sciences Center shows that yoga helps those with FS by increasing circulation to the limbs and releasing anxiety.

"[Yoganetics] has enriched my life and health. My fibromyalgia is 75 percent improved," says a woman who practices twice weekly.

Heart Disease

Yoga plays a key role in reversing heart disease, according to studies pioneered by Dean Ornish, M.D. His revolutionary approach combines a low-fat vegetarian diet, exercise, and an hour of daily yoga and meditation. According to the *American Journal of Cardiology,* 80 percent of patients eligible for bypass or angioplasty *avoided surgery* by following Ornish's program.

"So sure of yoga's health benefits are doctors at Cedars-Sinai Medical Center in Los Angeles that yoga is now an important part of their post-heart-attack program," says *U.S. News & World Report. Time* magazine reports that patients who participate in the yoga classes show "tremendous benefits," according to Dr. Noel Bairey Merz, the center's director—including lowered cholesterol and blood pressure, increased cardiovascular circulation, and reversal of artery blockage.

Hypertension

Yoga is effective in controlling high blood pressure, according to a clinical trial in India. Thirty-three people with hypertension, between the ages of thirty-five and sixty-five, were randomly divided into three groups. One group practiced yoga daily for eleven weeks, one group was given a daily drug, and the control group had no treatment. Both the yoga and pharmaceutical treatments were found to be effective in managing hypertension.

Stress

Stress underlies some 75 percent of doctor visits. Yoga has proven effective in stress management. Documented benefits include reductions in blood pressure, heart rate, respiration, and other stress indicators. (For more on stress, see chapter 2.)

Weight Loss

Research shows that using proper alignment in daily activities burns twice the calories we normally use, reports Arthur White, M.D. Alignment is a major emphasis of yoga training and translates to every moment of life. But weight loss is tied to *both* calorie usage and calorie consumption. Yoga plays a dual role in weight reduction by addressing the stress that underlies overeating. (For more on weight loss, see chapter 2.)

Notes

Preface

Burnett, Frances Hodgson. *The Secret Garden* (Boston: David R. Godine, 1987), 63.

Dürckheim, Karlfried Graf Von. *Hara: The Vital Centre of Man* (London: Mandala Books, 1977).

Hamilton, Linda, Ph.D. "The Dancers' Health Survey, Part I." *Dance Magazine,* November 1996, 57.

Rilke, Rainer Maria. *Letters to a Young Poet.* Translated by M. D. Herter Norton (New York: W. W. Norton & Co., Inc.), rev. 1954.

Introduction

Burnett, Frances Hodgson. *The Secret Garden* (Boston: David R. Godine, 1987), 198.

Price, Joan. "Brain Workouts for a Better Body." Copyright © 2001, Unconventional Moves. Internet: www.joanprice.com/articles/brainwrk.htm.

Chapter One

Lidell, Lucy. *The Sivananda Companion to Yoga* (New York: Simon & Schuster, 1983), 18.

MacDonald, George. *The Golden Key* (New York: Farrar, Straus & Giroux, 1967), 57.

Chapter Two

Bottom Line Personal. April 1, 1995, 8.

Corliss, Richard. "The Power of Yoga." *Time,* April 23, 2001, 60.

Feeney, Sheila Anne. "Protect Your Hearing, Because Once It Goes, It's Gone for Good." The *New York Daily News,* reprinted in the *Kansas City Star,* February 9, 1999.

Ina, Lauren. "It's Yoga." *Self,* July 1991, 109.

Nicolosi, Michelle. "Stretching before exercise . . . " *Orange County Register,* reprinted in the *Kansas City Star,* October 13, 1993.

Townley, Roderick. *The Great Good Thing* (New York: Atheneum, 2001), 93.

Wallis, Claudia. "Faith and Healing." *Time,* June 24, 1996, 59.

White, Arthur H., M.D., author interviews, June 1993.

Chapter Three

MacDonald, George. *At the Back of the North Wind* (New York: Children's Classics, 1990), 268.

Chapter Four

Anonymous. *The Eternal Verities* (Los Angeles: The Theosophy Company, 1940), 1–2.

Burnett, Frances Hodgson. *The Secret Garden* (Boston: David R. Godine, 1987), 148–149.

Frost, Robert. "The Road Not Taken," *The Poetry of Robert Frost* (New York: Holt, Rinehart & Winston, 1969), 105.
Ornish, Dean, M.D. *Dr. Dean Ornish's Program for Reversing Heart Disease* (New York: Random House, 1990), 168.
Todd, Mabel Elsworth. *The Thinking Body* (New York: Dance Horizons, 1937), 217–246; 284.
Van De Graaff, Kent. *Human Anatomy* (Dubuque, IA: William C. Brown, 1992).
Whitman, Walt. *Leaves of Grass* (New York: Doubleday, Doran & Co., Inc., 1940).

Chapter Five

Williams, Margery. *The Velveteen Rabbit* (New York: Doubleday & Co., Inc.), 17.

Chapter Six

Barrie, J. M. *Peter Pan* (Montreal: Tundra Books, 1988), 79.

Chapter Seven

MacDonald, George. *The Princess and the Goblin* (New York: Knopf, Everyman's Library, 1993), 162.

Chapter Eight

Baum, L. Frank. *The Wonderful Wizard of Oz* (New York: William Morrow & Company, 1899), 116.
Rasmussen, Eric, D.C., author interviews, June 1993.
White, Arthur H., M.D., author interviews, June 1993.

Chapter Nine

MacDonald, George. *The Golden Key* (New York: Farrar, Straus & Giroux, 1967), 59.

Chapter Ten

Dürckheim, Karlfried Graf Von. *Hara: The Vital Centre of Man* (London: Mandala Books, 1977), 108–109; 119; 138–139.
Eliot, T. S. *Four Quartets* (New York: Harcourt, Brace & Company, 1943), 17.
Saint-Exupéry, Antoine de. *The Little Prince* (New York: Harcourt Brace & World, 1943), 70.
Townley, Wyatt. *The Breathing Field: Meditations on Yoga*. Images by Eric Dinyer (Boston: Little, Brown & Company, Bulfinch Press), 2002.
White, E. B. *Charlotte's Web* (New York: Harper & Row, 1952), 183.

Health Guide

AIDS

Stukin, Stacie. "Health, Hope, and HIV." *Yoga Journal*, August 2001, 75–81.

Arthritis

Lipson, Elaine. "Yoga Works!" *Yoga Journal*, Winter 1999, 10.

Asthma

Lipson, Elaine. "Yoga Works!" *Yoga Journal*, Winter 1999, 10.

Back Pain

Klein, Arthur C., and Sobel, Dava. *Backache Relief* (New York: Penguin Books, 1986).

White, Arthur H., M.D., author interviews, June 1993.

Cancer

Colwell, Joanna. "Re-Examining Breast Health." *Yoga Journal,* October 2001, 96–103; 172.

Corliss, Richard. "The Power of Yoga." *Time,* April 23, 2001, 56–57.

Chronic Pain

Hyatt, Vicki T. "Minding Your Pain." *Yoga Journal,* October 2001, 35.

Depression

Powers, Ann. "American Influences Help Redefine the Practice of Yoga." *New York Times,* August 1, 2000.

Weintraub, Amy. "Better than Prozac?" *Yoga Journal,* August, 2001, 31.

Fibromyalgia

Lipson, Elaine. "Yoga Works!" *Yoga Journal,* Winter 1999, 12.

Heart Disease

Corliss, Richard. "The Power of Yoga." *Time,* April 23, 2001, 60–61.

Ornish, Dean, M.D. *Dr. Dean Ornish's Program for Reversing Heart Disease* (New York: Random House, 1990).

Hypertension

Murugesan, R., Govindarajulu, N., Bera, T. K. "Effect of Selected Yogic Practices on the Management of Hypertension." Internet: www.ncbi.nl. PubMed., National Library of Medicine.

Weight Loss

White, Arthur H., M.D., author interviews, June 1993.

To contact the author or learn more about Yoganetics classes,
workshops, appearances, videos, and books,
visit the Web site at
www.yoganetics.com.